ESCAPE AMERICA'S OVER-EATING EPIDEMIC

The AGE-Less Way

By

HELEN VLASSARA, MD

with

Sandra Woodruff, RD,

Jaime Uribarri, MD,

and

Gary E. Striker, MD

ISBN: 0615450040
ISBN-13: 9780615450049

Contents

Introduction

The Poly-Epidemic Puzzle

Why another book about food and health? Because we are not getting any healthier. Because we face far bigger problems now than before or at any other time in human history: several epidemics of major diseases that are all linked to modern food, which include diabetes, obesity, heart and kidney disease, Alzheimer's disease, and cancer. It's as though something in our food somehow continues to elude us.

For argument's sake, the elusive factor in these epidemics could be a group of harmful substances not previously linked to eating, i.e. Advanced Glycation End-products, or AGEs.

Based on more than forty years of research, myself and others have come to believe that AGEs, the subject of this book, are a known and serious, yet unsuspected player. Let us take a step back and consider the diseases we face today, starting with diabetes.

I was extremely fortunate early in my career to work side by side with some of the best minds in American medicine and science; they were blazing trails in diabetes and aging. We naively believed then, that diabetes would soon be cured, gone, history in another five years, ten at most. In fact, scientific advances since then have been slow. The outlook of diabetes and its many complications has been transformed and I am gratified to have personally contributed a few pieces of knowledge to that. But what about a cure? Well, the facts there are less glorious. Things have not gotten too far ahead on this score. Diabetes has surged instead into a worldwide epidemic.

As if this was not enough, other epidemics also emerged: obesity, heart disease, kidney disease, Alzheimer's, dementia, cancer, and many more. This "poly-epidemic" is extraordinarily unusual, particularly because it is not due to capricious viruses, resistant microbes or new gene mutations. The best and brightest in medicine and science have been unable to explain this turn of events, no matter how advanced and effective their research tools were.

Nevertheless, pieces of this poly-epidemic puzzle were coming together. For instance, many of these epidemics seemed to track closely with the phenomenon of larger body weight. Being heavy is as common now as it was before to be taller than our parents. Not only that, everyone today likely knows someone with diabetes, heart disease, or cancer: a family member, a friend, a neighbor. These diseases and health risks have become so widespread that they are seen everywhere. *Diabetic Living*, a magazine devoted to the disease, is not found only in doctors' waiting rooms, it can also be spotted at the supermarket next to *Glamour* and *House & Garden*. Nowadays, it is customary to see obese teenagers in t-shirts the size of small tents, eating pizza and drinking 64-ounce colas.

On a return trip from Europe, I was walking through the airport looking for my gate and was struck by the fact that Americans waiting to board a flight to New York were noticeably heavier than people waiting at gates to other parts of the world. Many of the New York–bound passengers were spilling over their seemingly too-narrow airport seats. What's more, it seems that we have accepted this new body shape, which is so different from the old image of the health-beaming, athletic American, an image that was envied and copied around the globe.

Has over-eating, an embarrassing personal trait, now become part of our character? If looks or pride do not count, what about the health and quality of life of us and our families? In this land of obsessive preoccupation with health, the latest drug discovery, organ transplants, customized medicine, stem cells and personal genomes, one in four of us is overeating to the point of being practically sick. Children today are so prone to obesity and its consequences that experts expect them to have a shorter lifespan than their parents. Yet, eighty percent of this is preventable by a moderate diet and more activity. There are plenty of diet books and exercise programs to choose from, so why is obesity still extremely prevalent?

Cultures change as societies evolve. Ours, if nothing else, is driven by technology and marketing. Food is cheaper and more abundant than ever before. Our eating behavior has also changed, along with other things. This, however, does not seem enough to explain the downward spiral of our health— eating more - presumably better - food should not necessarily be a cause of disease.

Cooking up trouble

Volumes are written about food and food processing. The discussion largely explores the industrial manipulation of nutrients and their sources—animals, plants or minerals—usually intended for purposes of production, preservation, transportation, and public consumption. Some arguments have condemned the intrusion of harmful chemicals, the excess of bad sugars or fats, and hormones in the food chain. Surely these have shed important new light. Even cooking has ignited some arguments. But why should cooking be a problem? The centuries-old practice of cooking over heat should carry the very stamp of safety.

It was only recently that it dawned on us to zero in on a clue that we had every reason to miss! Think of it: Our reflex response is to reach for the French fries, not mashed potatoes. Much of the allure of our Western diet comes from frying, grilling, and baking. This is certainly true for fast foods.

Why do we not go for uncooked food? For many reasons, including food safety. But the truth is that food *tastes* better when exposed to heat. Enhanced taste is often due to the unintended formation of AGEs. We have come to learn that AGEs are harmful oxidants. They are complex chemical substances made of sugars bound to proteins or fat. They naturally exist at low levels in all living organisms and have no ill effects. However, they can be toxic when present in excess. AGEs are normally controlled by our own antioxidants and other natural defenses. When oxidants build up and overwhelm these defenses, they cause damage. So when we cook foods by broiling or frying, we cook up trouble too. Since AGEs were a special focus of my team's research, we've known about the harmful effects of AGEs all along. Until recently, we were only interested in those AGEs that are produced in our body from our own major source of sugar (glucose). It was believed then that the quantity of AGEs became dangerous only when sugar got out of control, as in diabetes, or in older age.

> ◎ *The acronym AGEs was actually coined to remind us that AGEs are linked to the ills of aging and that their presence in diabetes is responsible for the accelerated aging that is part of this and other chronic diseases.*

We thought that we had all the pieces to the puzzle, except that we kept missing a crucial piece, which was that most AGEs arise from our food. Another piece we failed to notice was that over the past several decades, our diet has undergone a dramatic transformation, shifting from fresh homemade foods to largely commercially prepared fare, or what we now refer to as the typical Western or American diet.

Around the turn of the twentieth century, food chemists had identified AGEs as substances that enhance food flavors, smells, and color. Since taste in food is the ticket to profit for the food industry, it need not be doubted that most commercially prepared food products would be packed with increasing amounts of AGEs. No time was wasted as consumers now had countless choices of tasty foods to eat. People began stocking grocery carts with large-sized packages filled with new gustatory pleasures, and a new era of food consumerism in America began. This new era of a food-for-profit industry and of unprecedented overeating in America rapidly spread to the entire globe. Just consider all those developments that are no longer strange or even novel: the huge food portions, the sprawling supermarkets and restaurant chains, the profusion of commercial food products, and the huge industry of food advertising in daily life. Based on our latest data, bacon, burgers, pizzas, chips, hot dogs, and snack foods, all American favorites, are steeped in AGEs. The overeating frenzy is in full swing, and it will not be stopped so easily.

Since AGEs are natural substances, it was not easy to nail down this new tenuous link between health and food AGEs. It took many more years of studying laboratory animals to be convinced that cutting down AGEs in daily food could in fact prevent or arrest these diseases.

An extra tip at the time was the possibility that this simple cutting of AGEs could work wonders without cutting down calories—in other words, without going hungry - a most unexpected and nearly as exciting finding!

In Harm's Way

There was work to be done. The very next step was to find out about food AGEs in human health. We already knew that AGEs are a matter of concern for those who have diabetes, or the elderly. What we did not suspect then was that young healthy people would turn out to have alarming levels of AGEs in their blood too. These AGEs turned out to originate from the standard American diet, as broiled steaks, fried chicken, bacon, fries and such, a diet rich in toxic AGEs. This fact was never seriously considered before.

A striking realization throughout these studies was that food AGE intake went hand in hand with inflammatory markers, and that this occurred in people of all ages. Inflammation has long been known to underlie most chronic diseases. This could mean that persons who habitually consume AGE-rich diets (i.e. most of us!) run the risk of prematurely exhausting their natural defenses. We then made the prediction that frequent consumption of AGE-rich foods, not only lures us toward overeating - and obesity - but at the same time, makes us vulnerable to diseases, of which diabetes is a prime example.

Within a couple of years, we found that people eating AGE-rich foods were more likely to have pre-diabetes (or insulin-resistance), making it also more likely for them to develop high blood pressure, and heart or kidney disease. They were, in other words, in harm's way. First reports of these findings prompted a storm of interest and debates in the United States and around the world. A few years later, helped by funds from a prestigious national award, our suspicions were confirmed. AGEs in favorite American foods work as potent oxidants, and when they are over-consumed, can deplete native antioxidants. As a result, over-consumption of appetizing AGE-rich foods brings us ever closer toward obesity and disease.

Just as important, this was true for people too young for these problems. Newborn infants even can take up way too many AGEs from the mother's blood as well as from heat-processed infant formulas. Infant foods contain up to several hundred times more AGEs than breast milk or food prepared at home. This little-known fact could partly account for children's higher rates of diseases previously seen only in older adults.

More pieces of the puzzle gradually fell into place. Not only persons with diabetes, but others with kidney or heart disease also have too many AGEs in their blood.

Another fascinating association emerged between brain function in "healthy" older people and AGEs. That is, the higher the AGE levels are in their blood, the faster the rate at which memory and attention span deteriorates, and the worse the residual brain damage will be after a stroke.

People with high AGE blood levels are also likely to have too many AGEs in their skin. When this happens, the skin becomes less elastic, which can lead to wrinkles and sagging. Another problem that comes along with excess AGEs is a reduced ability of the skin to repair itself and heal smoothly without leaving scars.

Incidentally, AGEs—proven to be toxic to many types of cells—may also play an important role in the development of certain common tumors. This may be one reason that patients with diabetes and various chronic diseases have a higher propensity toward certain types of cancer.

A Battle We Can Win

In spite of these discouraging facts, there is exciting news. As people adopted the AGE-Less Way, regardless of chronological age or health status, indicators of inflammation and disease all plummeted to normal levels. Many also realized substantial benefits. Blood glucose, insulin, blood lipids, and often body weight all improved in a matter of weeks or months. All this was done by simply switching meal preparation methods to those that hinder AGEs, or by avoiding foods too rich in these oxidants like junk food. Very importantly, calorie intake remained the same. That is the centerpiece of the AGE-Less Way and a sharp difference from most diet programs. AGE-Less means staying healthy and youthful; it does *not* mean going hungry.

The AGE-Less Way is not just another diet gimmick. AGEs have managed to evade suspicion and bypass all conventional wisdom, but we have now recognized their importance and harmful effects. AGEs are the perfect "double deal": They make food ever more appealing, and little by little rob us of our treasured health. Therefore, reducing the amount of AGEs consumed, while maintaining caloric intake, is sure to improve the odds.

The existence and nature of AGEs remain largely unknown to the general public—and, for that matter, to many health care professionals. Translating research into clinical practice is notoriously slow in the medical community, even in today's information-obsessed world. Meanwhile, countless accounts spell out our predicament: We may now live longer, but in poorer health. We are told that this trend is not - cannot be - right. Most of us admit that our collective eating habits have changed dramatically in the last two generations, and not for the better. Our health matters. If each of us does not protect it, who will?

One intention of this book is to open this subject up for an honest conversation. It is time to become more aware of the ways corporate food industry weigh in on decisions and policies that end up supporting the decline, rather than the improvement of our health. This book addresses an unconscious folly involved in choosing to turn a blind eye to things we may not like to face: the fact that a great majority of us willingly and avidly ingest toxins. Many might be moved to wonder how it is that we acquiesced to this major "tampering" with our food supply or why we surrendered our own and our family's entitlement to health in the process. Hopefully, many will want to know how we can reclaim these rights.

The other intention is precisely to examine how to control AGEs, here and now. By reducing the consumption of these toxins, we can sidestep serious health problems. If food AGEs strike you as just one more piece of bad news that is encroaching upon your lifestyle today, think of it this way: this is a problem, but a problem you can easily and totally control at no extra cost. The knowledge and skills are available. If you have the will, this book can help you make changes that last and truly matter to your health. This is no small bargain.

The AGE-Less Way

As is obvious by now, this is not a traditional diet book. The focus of the AGE-Less Way is to put a stop to a real folly and how to avert or reverse serious trouble. Following this program helps restore natural strength and reduces vulnerability to disease. It is wholly centered on core health and the belief that all else flows from this strong base.

The AGE-Less Way can also speed up weight loss. If your goal is to produce faster and longer lasting results, you can combine the AGE-Less principles with just about any eating plan. The AGE-Less Way is really about improving health from the inside out and adding years of good health to your life.

You may be tempted to skip ahead to the last chapters of this book, to the eating plan and recipes. However, we encourage you to read the first part of the book, where we dig up the hidden story of AGEs, what they really are, where they come from, and the many liberties they take with your health. This completely new understanding will give you a unique framework to build your own rationale on why you should make a change in your life.

New does not mean difficult. You will find out that the AGE-Less Way is much simpler to follow than most dietary plans. You do not have to pay for expensive products or gadgets, or make complicated recipes with hard-to-find ingredients. Better yet, we promise that you will never feel hungry. You can apply the AGE-Less Way principles even when dining away from home. The AGE-Less Way does not advocate severe calorie restriction nor does it favor some nutrients, such as carbohydrates or proteins, at the expense of others. It is no big secret that weight-loss diets by themselves do not work that well in the long run. The AGE-Less Way does work, especially for older adults when cutting too many calories is neither advisable nor sustainable. There is a wealth of science in this book, as well as case studies of people like you, with or without diabetes or other common conditions.

No matter what your age or your current health status is, the AGE-Less Way will work for you. The payoff is not just a trimmer waistline; it is a better core health, a clearer mind, and a longer, more vibrant life.

Acknowledgments

This book is based on the vision and foresight of many prominent scientists who first recognized that AGEs are substances with enormous health implications. The flow of scientific information sadly is slow and unwieldy, since translating complex chemical phenomena is difficult. To then attempt to apply this knowledge in a way that makes it accessible to all is a real challenge. This is not a unique problem. It took several centuries for Galileo's discoveries to be incorporated in the collective knowledge. Pertinent to this book, it took exactly a century for the simple chemical reaction discovered by Louis Camille Maillard to become first immensely popular and then, to unravel. By now, AGEs and their *bitter-sweet* implications touch everyone's life. This book aims to make up for some of the lost time.

Writing it has been a challenging and rejuvenating journey. Putting the AGE-Less Way together took nearly forty years of relentless examination, discovery and failure, but also gave back enormous gratification. My personal gratitude goes to the mentors who unselfishly shared their inspiration and those who offered undiluted faith and enthusiastic support. Deep thanks go to the countless collaborators throughout the international scientific community who embraced these ideas with open minds.

The lion's share of this work is dedicated to the team of close colleagues, scientists, clinicians, clinical research coordinators, hospital staff, experts in nutrition, dietetics, statistics, and especially my co-authors, who persevered through thick and thin for many years—and continue to this very day. For, they too know, our work is yet to be done.

PART 1:

Why We Over-Eat

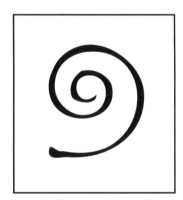

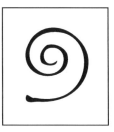

Chapter 1:
The Food Debacle
of the 20th Century

Our health is intricately tied to the amount of food we consume and the nutrients in it. Despite vastly improved nutrition, more people in this country die from diseases connected to diet than at any other time in history. The sheer quantity and variety of foods available to us are partly to blame; we can eat as much as we like as often as we like, which surely has contributed to the current obesity epidemic. Food components like cholesterol, trans fats, and sugar have been directly implicated in certain diseases. But these do not tell the whole story.

Our research points to a completely different but major issue that has not been addressed yet—specifically, the presence of oxidants in food. We have heard a lot about oxidants that cause the generation of free radicals in the body. Normally, they are dealt with by powerful antioxidant mechanisms. Yet, when they are present in excess, they can overwhelm these defenses. Too many free radicals work against us, causing disease and faster aging. Up to now, they were thought of as something that affects us only later in life, after decades of exposure. We now know that they are everywhere around us, especially in our food, continuously causing damage that accumulates over time. New evidence points out that there is such an abundance of oxidants coming in with our food that our antioxidants have no chance to be effective. This may account for the fact that oral antioxidants are ineffective in preventing disease.

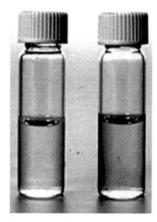

Figure 1: Vials containing water and egg-white (shown on the left), or egg-white plus sugar (on the right). The darker (actually, yellow-brown) color that appears after a couple of weeks in the right vial is due to AGE formation. The dark liquid also has a familiar flavor and aroma, as in caramel. This is also due to AGEs.

Among the most important oxidants is a class of compounds called advanced glycation endproducts, or AGEs for short. They are commonly referred to as glycotoxins. You might be surprised to know that AGEs are quite familiar to our senses; they impart flavor, color, and aroma to our food when heat is applied during cooking. The body's defenses can neutralize these oxidants as long as they are not present in excess amounts. As we will see, AGEs do have good features, but it is their excess that makes them toxic. Being that AGEs look, taste and smell good, their use is widespread in modern foods, which makes it easy for us to over-eat and for them to build up to toxic levels in our tissues. That is when they cause trouble in the form of diabetes, as well as heart, brain or kidney disease. AGEs make us age before our time. AGEs can indeed affect health in many and profound ways. Sadly, this trend has now spread to the younger generations, causing diabetes and obesity in children. Let's begin by examining what AGEs are.

A Discovery and a Blind Spot

To get a first hand idea of how AGEs form, we can try a simple experiment. All you have to do is fill a small clear glass bottle with water, and then add a tablespoon of sugar and one egg white. Close the bottle tightly and let it sit at room temperature for a week or two. The liquid will slowly become opaque as it goes from colorless to yellow, gold, orange, and finally brown (**Figure 1**). The change in color is an indicator of a chemical reaction between sugar and protein that produces new substances called advanced glycation end-products (AGEs).

These can also form in food. You can see this happen every day to bread in your toaster.

Amazing as it sounds, this same process happens in your body all the time. Small amounts of AGEs form as metabolic byproducts from a chemical process that links sugars to proteins, fats (lipids), or DNA, and the body has mechanisms to remove them. The AGEs that arise from the body's own sugars, proteins, lipids, and so on, develop slowly, over weeks or months. Some are only transiently present and may be short-lived, while others form free radicals and cause oxidation (a process similar to rusting). Some are colorful or even fluorescent. There can be literally hundreds of different types of AGE compounds in the body and in the food supply. For simplicity's sake, scientists have collected all of them under a single umbrella—namely AGEs.

It is only in the past forty years or so that researchers recognized the profound effects that AGEs can have on health and disease, and few suspected that food AGEs could be toxic. Although we knew that AGEs were linked to aging and diabetes, we believed that they were formed exclusively inside the body from glucose, the most abundant sugar in our blood and tissues.

The process of glycation begins as glucose latches onto certain amino acids. Whether or not AGEs will eventually form depends on the local conditions, such as the levels of glucose, and the type of proteins or lipids nearby. Once they gather in quantity, AGEs can damage proteins or fats and many body structures in a number of ways (**Table 1-1**). However, since it was believed that AGEs form principally in the body, and at a very slow rate, there was little concern, except when glucose was high, as in diabetes, or much later in life.

When the news broke out that the majority of AGEs in the body could come from food, there was disbelief, as is often the case with any new paradigm. Gathering definitive proof on the negative health implications of food AGEs took years of study. During this process, a blind spot came into full view— specifically, that AGEs in food could be harmful and even a primary source of AGEs in the body.

Table 1 -1: How AGEs Affect Us

- Change the way proteins, fats, nucleic acids work
- Generate too many Free Radicals = Increase Oxidation
- Decrease our anti-Oxidant Defenses = Oxidant Stress
- Aggravate our Immune system = cause Inflammation
- Damage insulin-producing cells = Type 1 Diabetes
- Cause Insulin Resistance = Type 2 Diabetes
- Build up Abdominal Fat = Increase Body Weight
- Increase "Bad' Cholesterol in arteries = Block blood flow to vital organs
- Build rigid bridges between collagen proteins = harden arteries, joints, tendons, cause lens cataracts, wrinkled skin

---

The Origins

For thousands of years, humans have been cooking our food over a fire—if not directly, then indirectly, via an array of tools and techniques that use some sort of heat source. There is no question that at the moment our ancestors discovered fire, they took a major, decisive step toward survival and secured our place as the most successful mammal on earth.

What they discovered early on is that after eating from a hunting or scavenging expedition, the scraps of leftover meat kept far better and longer if passed over fire or smoke. Also at this time, people realized the importance of shelf life and storage of foods. What else was imparted by fire? That's right: AGEs! While cooking helped preserve food, it also generated AGEs. Our food taste preferences slowly developed along these same lines, incorporating other empirical observations, such as the effect of salt, sugar, and fat. No other species developed cooking skills. As these abilities passed from generation to generation over thousands of years, they helped humans survive, migrate and spread across the continents. From an evolutionary perspective, we can say that cooking with fire helped us prosper as a species. However, the excessive amount of AGEs we consume today may do more harm than good (**Figure 2**).

Food chemists have known about AGEs for more than one hundred years. They were first identified by Louis-Camille Maillard, a French food chemist. He called them "browning products" because of their golden-brown appearance on the surface of baked and fried foods. Food chemists were the first to adopt Maillard's discoveries, when they realized that the rich flavors and enticing aromas associated with cooking were actually due to AGEs. In the subsequent years, food manufacturers developed new ways to optimize the conditions and levels of AGEs in foods in order to improve their taste.

This is not an indictment of the food industry, since AGEs have many positive qualities in the right amounts. It is hard to ignore that heating made food safer for storage and more digestible. For a very long time no one took notice of the fact that AGEs in food had ill health effects. It is only recently that we've begun to understand the negative health effects of over-consumption of AGEs in food.

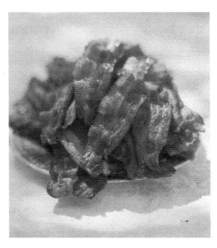

Figure 2: Fried bacon, a favorite American food is the No. 1 AGE-richest item. In just 5 minutes (with no oil added) you can have several days' AGE allowance in a single serving. Worse yet, much of it ends up in your arteries.

The Good and the Bad

Although they add shelf-life and taste to foods, AGEs can have major negative effects. When present in excess amounts, they act as oxidants creating harmful free radicals. AGEs can chemically alter the building blocks of our genetic material such as DNA. They can cause inflammation since the body reacts to AGEs as if they were "foreign," much like bacteria.

AGEs can also act as adhesive material; they stick to different proteins or bind them together like glue. Lipoproteins, the fat-carrying proteins that circulate in our blood, also known as blood cholesterol, can attract sugar to form new AGEs, or may bind precursors of AGEs that come in with food. This makes lipoproteins sticky, a reason for which they end up plugging our arteries. These are only a few of the deleterious properties of AGEs that hasten not only one disease, but the entire aging process (**Table 1-1**).

As lipoproteins are oxidized, they form patches inside the blood vessels that resemble rust on the inside of old metal pipes. This rusty layer causes blood vessels to narrow or become blocked. As a result, tissues and organs do not receive adequate blood—and oxygen. In the heart, this can lead to heart failure or a heart attack; in the brain it may cause a stroke; and in the legs it leads to cramping (especially during walking or exercise), open ulcers, or even the loss of a limb.

By forming rigid bridges between adjacent proteins, AGEs can cause stiffness or brittleness in bones, joints and tendons. Here is what happens when AGEs attach to collagen, the long fibers that hold our tissues together. These fibers normally slide past each other, like smooth ropes. This allows bending and movement. However, if the fibers become welded together by AGEs, muscles, tendons, and joints are no longer as flexible. This is easy to see in older persons. Since they tend to have higher AGE levels, they generally have difficulty stretching their joints or bending their back.

As with proteins, fats can also be modified by AGEs, although this is normally a slow process. But fats from processed food may already be oxidized and "rusty". As a result, they're very sticky. The first stop for the sticky oxidized fat that is absorbed from the digestive tract is the abdomen. Did you ever wonder why we tend to store fat from fried foods around our middles? Now you know. The more tasty, crusty AGE-modified fats we eat, the more abdominal fat we gain. Sometimes we may not even see it yet because they hide deep inside the abdomen. Therefore, an expanding waist line is a sure risk factor for heart disease or diabetes.

Chapter 2:
The Missing Link

Around the middle of the twentieth century, the first warning signs of a rise in debilitating diseases, such as heart disease, diabetes and obesity, emerged. Various schools of thought ensued, unanimously linking them to food, and by turns, to too much protein, fat, or carbohydrates.

After the bad rap was given to "bad" fats, there was a shift away from saturated fats. However, since the incidence of obesity and heart disease continued to rise, saturated fats hardly seemed to be the whole story. Then came the trans fats. Fortunately, those dangerous lipids are now removed from the grocery shelf. Processed "hydrogenated" oils are full of oxidized lipids. Fat of all kinds in food is easily oxidized, and this fuels the formation of AGEs. It follows that, during heat processing or cooking, AGEs are far more rapidly generated on both fats and adjacent proteins. Therefore, AGE-bound fat could well be how some fats got their bad name. While fats would be far less harmful if consumed in their natural state, free of AGEs or other oxidants, they are almost never eaten this way. Even air or light can oxidize fats — you are certainly familiar with how easily butter becomes "rancid" as it oxidizes. By now you can probably guess that many of the benefits of even "healthful" fats, for instance of omega-3s, are easily lost during cooking. This is due to the formation of new AGEs, which robs them of their "good" properties.

Diets based on carbohydrate over-consumption actually increase body weight. Beyond that, little thought has gone into the well known fact that some sugars, especially fructose, form AGEs with proteins and fats during food processing and cooking, or what happens after they are absorbed inside the body. Fructose is abundant in a great number of modern foods and drinks and can form AGEs ten times faster than glucose.

Connecting the Dots

It is no secret that the epidemic of obesity has not been stopped by low-fat foods, low-carb diets, or meatless Mondays. Although many dieters have had success losing weight following these approaches, most have found it very difficult to stick to them over time—and even some of those who can keep up the diets find it difficult to shed the pounds.

According to the Center for Disease Control, between 1960 and 1970 the U.S. population gained about 1% in body mass index (BMI), from 24.3 to 25.4. Body mass index is essentially a measurement which takes both height and weight into account. This change in BMI is plausible. But what seems hard to comprehend is that Americans gained another 8% in the subsequent decade (BMI increased to 33.3). This sudden and huge leap toward gross obesity occurred in all age groups, and it is still increasing. Twice as many children are obese today than at the end of the twentieth century. Along with obesity came an increased incidence of diabetes, high blood pressure, and heart disease. What is it that caused such a rapid change in our lives from robust health to these pandemics? Is it just calories? It can't be because not all those affected by these diseases are obese. Furthermore, many who are slightly overweight are now falling prey to these diseases at a younger age.

As we touched on above, new evidence has been alerting us to the possibility that AGEs in food could well be what stirs this cycle of chronic disease and obesity. Since specialized AGE-tests are still not widely available, this crucial link has largely gone unnoticed by health care providers. Perhaps there are other reasons for this lack of attention to a role for AGEs as agents of harm – such as intentional dismissal, competing interests and many others less benign. Nonetheless, the data seem as easy as connecting the dots: the levels of AGEs in the blood of healthy persons go hand in hand with BMI. That is, those with the highest BMI also have the highest levels of AGEs. Correlations between BMI and AGE levels in the body remain significant even after adjusting for the obvious players, such as calories, fat, or gender and age. In other words, with respect to weight gain and weight related problems, AGEs are a very significant and important factor. Those who indulge in high-AGE foods, such as baked or fried goods and fast foods, are more likely to have more body fat for a given number of calories consumed than those who prefer foods prepared by stewing, poaching, or steaming, all of which are lower in AGEs.

In other words,

 ...tasty AGEs drive us to over-eat, especially AGE-rich foods. But they also can make us retain body fat that is not usable for energy. This makes it easier to understand why over the years we put on weight even when we do not over-eat.

When Defense Turns Into Offense

We humans come with a defensive mechanism that helps overcome danger inside our body. This process is known as the inflammatory (or immune) response. It employs an army of "bodyguards" called white blood cells that are ready to protect us. They do not allow foreigners to trespass our borders. Lymphocytes and macrophages (working like "Pac Men") will attack, kill the invaders and remove damaged cells or tissues. These actions constitute what is generally called inflammation. It is recognized by the typical symptoms it produces: pain, redness, pus, fever, cough, and more. These symptoms usually go away as healing is completed. But, like any drawn out stressful state, especially if prolonged, inflammation can take a toll on health. As a matter of fact, such chronic, low-grade inflammation lurks beneath – even precedes – a host of common health problems, ranging from heart disease and obesity to diabetes and aging. This has been known for a long time, but its origin has remained elusive.

Scientists thought, for instance, that the normal wear and tear of the body generates too many free radicals, and it is this excess that causes oxidation and inflammation. Yet, there is an increasing consensus that free radicals are only part of the problem. Chronic inflammation needs to draw from a large and sustained source of oxidants. What can this source be? AGEs have long been among the candidates, since they accumulate in the body over a lifetime and are biologically capable of stirring up inflammation. Food AGEs are an even more plausible source, since they come into the body already-made, constantly and in a great excess.

Quite possibly, as AGEs then begin to pile up in tissues, a defensive response to get rid of them is mounted. Since new AGEs keep pouring in daily, this ordinarily silent process eventually turns into a chronic inflammatory state, which is harmful. Food AGEs could well be what turns normal self-defense into offense. Over-consumption of AGE-rich foods could then be among the initiators of the current epidemics, or represents a common ingredient and missing link.

This concept has now been confirmed in clinical studies of over five hundred healthy persons. The blood level of AGEs was directly linked to the AGEs consumed with their food. Many participants had inflammation in proportion to the AGEs in their diet. Inflammatory substances, also called cytokines, fluctuated along with the AGEs consumed with meals. This was alarming news to these volunteers, since by their own account they were healthy. None of them suspected that they might run a risk for diabetes or heart disease. It was a wake up call.

Beating them at their Own Game

Fortunately, the moment came when these fears were alleviated. A new clinical study helped establish a practical way to get around this problem. It was conducted in about seventy volunteers with high blood AGE levels. Blood AGE levels are normally around 6-10 units (U) per milliliter (ml) of blood; in these volunteers they averaged at about 15 U/ml. Half of the volunteers were placed on the AGE-Less Way program (described in detail in Parts 2 and 3) for four months. Their caloric intake was kept at levels that were identical to their routine diet (2,000 kcal/day on average), but their AGE intake with food was trimmed to about half their normal intake, which was around 15,000 kilo units (kU) of AGE per day. To avoid confusion later on, you may note here that, when referring to AGEs in the blood, we talk about *Units (U)*, while for foods we use *kilo units (kU)*.

After about four months on the AGE-Less Way, the levels of AGEs in their blood decreased by about one third. In other words, the levels of blood AGEs decreased from 15 to 10 U/ml. In addition, there was a large drop (about 50%) in levels of inflammatory markers and oxidants in these volunteers, compared to those kept on their usual diet. A key here is to understand that there was no change in calories or nutrients consumed by either group. So, blood AGEs could not be tied to the amount of food they ate. Only to the way meals were prepared.

What can be taken away from these studies? First, the marked improvement in inflammation after the AGE-Less Way program meant that these volunteers had inflammation from the start. Second, this inflammatory situation had to be related to the AGEs present in their everyday diet, since it subsided after being on the AGE-Less Way program.

From this study, we surmised that the amount of AGEs consumed by many "healthy" adults – anywhere from 15,000 kU and upward - is unhealthy. It is at least twice what it should be. The safe range of AGE consumption –where inflammation is not detectable - is around or below 8,000 AGE kU/day. We will discuss this in greater detail later, but an important take-home message here is that reducing AGEs to this safe range takes no more than a few months. The best part yet - a real bonus - is that this can be achieved without sacrificing useful nutrients or feeling low in energy. You can beat AGEs at their own game, without throwing away "the baby with the bathwater."

Chapter 3:
Food for Profit

Ubiquitous and Alluring

Anyone who has ever toasted bread or roasted meat in his or her own kitchen has seen AGE formation in action. You cannot miss the changes in color and consistency, as the surface of bread or meat becomes golden, then brown and crusty. In the case of meat, it becomes thick and caramel-like and, if you wait long enough, or if you brush it with a layer of honey, it will become dark, or even black with a solid and crunchy texture. Other foods turn to shades of golden-brown, covered by a crispy, brittle and, alas, a wonderfully flavorful surface.

While new AGEs will form when food is just warmed up, many more will form – and faster - at high temperatures. For instance, the temperature reached by steaming or poaching will not exceed 212 degrees Fahrenheit, but baking or grilling can reach temperatures that are more than twice as high. This simply means that the higher the heat and the longer the cooking time, the more AGEs are formed.

Few can resist the smell of freshly cooked food. We respond to these odors in many ways. We experience a pleasant, familiar, comforting feeling as we begin to feel hungry. The pleasant scents and flavors come from volatile AGEs, and admittedly these are what we love about food. They can instantly bring us back to our earliest and most intense memories.

While humans have cooked their foods for thousands of years, the epidemic diseases tied to food have surged only in the past fifty or so years. Part of this is explained, as we noted in the last chapter, by the fact that we live longer and have easy access to more food. But that is not the only explanation.

AGEs became commercially valuable when it was realized that AGEs add delicious smell and taste to foods. Since it was not known that AGEs could be toxic, the food industry began manufacturing products that contained AGEs. Cheaper methods were devised for processing food and with more tasty AGEs in it. Mass production, storing, and distributing food became infinitely more profitable as nutrients became less perishable. Dry-heat sterilization does not only solve the practical aspects of shelf-life, it also offers better taste, due to the higher AGEs content. Food chemists eventually figured out that there is endless room for different combinations of chemically produced flavors that imitate natural flavors. Many of these are artificially synthesized AGEs. Marketing and advertising have taken on the task of shaping our tastes for food AGEs. Needless to say, food sells best if it contains lots of AGEs, even if it has little else to offer.

A Canadian study suggested that about ninety percent of "fun food" offered to children is of poor nutritional quality. Studies such as this did not consider AGEs. If they did, they would find that fun foods are all sources of AGEs. This is not meant to downplay the importance of known contaminants. The only point is that AGEs represent a far greater hazard than is realized.

> *"…The story of how …what to eat ever got so complicated reveals a great deal about the imperatives of food industry, nutrition science and – ahem – journalism, three parties that stand to gain much from widespread confusion surrounding the most elemental question.." M. Pollan, In Defense of Food", NY, 2008*

For example, almost everyone knows that sweetened colas are bad, since too much sugar can cause obesity, diabetes, and vascular disease. Therefore, staying away from them is a good idea. What is not realized is that what draws us to these drinks is not just the sweet taste of sugar, but the taste of AGEs. Many consumers switch to diet cola as a healthier substitute, since it provides a similar taste without the added sugar. According to the labels, there are no calories in artificial sweeteners; hence these drinks are thought to be safe for dieters.

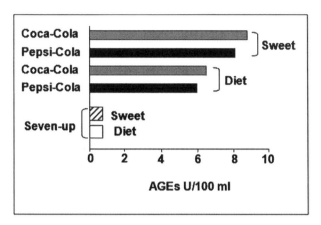

Figure 3: More AGEs are present in brown-color drinks (like in *colas*) than in clear drinks. Dark color drinks have about the same AGEs, whether they are artificially sweetened or not, marked as "diet". So sugar is not the only problem with these drinks. The message here is that, "diet" colas may not be much safer.

What is not printed on the label is that brown colored diet sodas contain nearly the same amount of AGEs as non-diet dark sodas (**Figure 3**), which is why the taste is similar to their sweet cousins. The dark color and characteristic flavor are due to AGEs that are pre-made by caramelizing (heating) sugars, such as fructose, which is ten times more effective than glucose in generating AGEs. Here is something else you should know: they can generate many more new AGEs as they react with food proteins or fats in our digestive tract. So, in this respect, diet colas are not much safer than non-diet varieties.

The consumption of sweetened soft drinks has caused an epidemic of pre-diabetes in children and adolescents. For instance, sugar-sweetened beverages and fruit juices represent up to 15% of the total calories consumed by children and make a big contribution to obesity in this age group. Since colas, unlike fruit juices, contain AGEs, they are also an unsuspected source of toxins. AGEs in colas are cheap to make and can be packaged in huge, colorful bottles of ever-increasing size that are sold at lower and lower prices.

Eating Over-Drive

If AGEs can cause diseases, why can't we ban them or simply avoid them? Some answers to this question may be obvious, but they would be economically and politically difficult to enact.

As we have seen, one answer is simply the ubiquitous nature of AGE-laden processed foods. These foods are cheap and readily available. The name, junk food, attached to them says it all. But low cost cannot be the only explanation for overeating; it would be even less expensive if we ate less. Hunger is not the only factor that drives eating; it is also the desire for the taste of food and the satisfaction of eating. Almost all of us live in a state of over-eating, a real folly when you think of it. AGEs seem to be in the driver's seat, spurring the appetite, urging us to reach for more food than is needed. It is almost as if eating AGEs causes us to crave more AGEs. In short, we may be addicted to AGE-laden food. There is no hard evidence yet that AGEs are addictive. However, we are at an important cross-roads: News agencies have been announcing the peculiar "addictive" properties of processed, high-corn syrup or fatty foods in animals and the changes in the brain's responses to AGE-rich foods identified in obese persons. The phenomena of ceaseless eating, craving or snacking and the deep discomfort many people experience with dieting suggests that there is something about our food that causes a craving that cannot be satisfied with fruits and vegetables, not even when sugar or salt are added to them.

Even without consuming too many extra calories, we still take in an amount of AGEs far greater than what our body can handle safely. While clinical studies show that the ingestion of about 5000-8000 kU per day of food AGEs can be handled by a healthy adult, the average consumption, at least in the state of New York, is about 15,000 kU/day and often above 40,000 kU/day. This high AGE intake is related to the way food is prepared, not necessarily to the types or the amount of food consumed. Frequent intake of an excess of AGEs can cause increased oxidative stress, inflammation, and eventually leads to disease. We need to take a hard look at this fact and realize the risk – to us and to our family - involved in ignoring it.

A Vicious Cycle

A very important clue is weight gain of any degree, not only the more extreme form of obesity, since it comes with inflammation that affects our arteries, heart and brain. That means that gaining fat is like developing a low-grade fever. Too many fat-filled cells get into a state of distress. If the amount of added fat is too large, the smoldering inflammation becomes chronic. This inflammation interferes with the work that insulin has to do and causes a condition called *insulin resistance*. Over time, this can cause high blood sugar, diabetes or heart problems.

Fat in cooked or processed food comes into the body already modified by AGEs (AGE-fat). AGE-fat is not very useful for our energy needs because it is not easily metabolized. Therefore, it tends to sit inside fat cells in the abdomen, like a lump. But AGE-fat is not just dead weight, as it stirs up inflammation that affects our arteries, heart, or brain.

Let us see how the unhealthy side of food AGEs was discovered. Researchers who study diabetes or heart disease use laboratory animals traditionally fed a standardized processed diet that has saturated or "bad" fat added to it. This diet would be like adding fried bacon to a broiled hamburger, making it super high in AGEs (let's call this food AGE-rich). Laboratory mice eating this diet predictably develop obesity, diabetes, and severe vascular disease. However, if the time it took to cook this fatty diet was less (say, for 5 minutes instead of 15 minutes), it contained far fewer AGEs. It actually becomes an AGE-Less food. Amazingly enough, mice that ate AGE-Less food gained less weight than those who were fed the AGE-rich diet, even if they ate exactly the same amount of fat. Even more amazing, only the mice that ate the AGE-rich food developed diabetes and vascular disease.

Another striking aspect of these remarkable findings in animals is that they were very similar to, and told a great deal about us, humans, as we will see below. The advantage of studying animals is that it is easier to get a deeper understanding about diseases because these progress at a much faster rate in animals with shorter lives than humans.

What can one take away from these studies? First, not all fat is bad, an important point since we cannot live without it. Second, non heat-processed fat could be much less harmful, since it would then contain fewer AGEs. The fat we consume today comes from already heat-processed sources and contain large amounts of oxidant AGEs that can increase even more when we cook them. Since most of us consume more fat than we should, we should keep in mind that we also ingest plenty of AGE-fat. Third, since the facts stated in various nutrition manuals and labels are based on food in its natural state (i.e. fresh), they tell us neither the whole story nor the right one. Most foods are consumed neither raw nor fresh. Rather, they are heat-processed in one way or another, which almost always guarantees that they are rich in AGEs. So food labels tell only part – possibly not the most useful - of the story.

Indeed, the most effective way to add bad fat to your body is by consuming food rich in AGE-fat. That kind of fat is extremely abundant in red meats, pizzas, bacon, cheeses, butter, and so on. Outside of fat itself, frequent binging on these delicious foods will add to your body load of AGEs and will increase inflammation. Since fat and AGEs are almost always bound together, consuming too much processed fat is the worst case scenario. Plus, AGE-fat is difficult to lose, which explains why it is so easy to gain weight even when the intake is modest. Therefore, we need a plan to revise our eating habits since our health is on the balance.

The new fact is that fatness, insulin resistance, and diabetes are all linked to food by AGE-fat – not just plain fat.

Getting Around an Addiction

You may be wondering by now, is it possible to exchange our old habits for new ones even if they are healthier? In this day and age with the availability of a fast food chain on every block, it may seem difficult. Based on the experience of hundreds of healthy people, we can assure you the answer is yes, positively yes. There are many encouraging successful examples on similar grounds. Consider the popularity of sugar substitutes, of less fatty meals, of turkey-burgers or veggies. People of all ages, particularly the young, are now opting for water or fresh juices, rather than sugary dark colas. Think of cigarette smoking, a terrible addiction that cost millions of lives, but which has been successfully conquered by a great many people. Above all, it is much easier to exchange unsafe eating habits with safer ones, especially if they can be equally satisfying. Fortunately, the AGE-Less Way is generous and rewarding. It does not require going hungry, since the amount or type of food does not have to be changed, unless it is necessary.

We can guess what you might be thinking: "I've already cut back on fat, sugar, and salt. Do I now have to give up foods just because they *taste good*?" Definitely not! Quite the opposite! You will find that The AGE-Less Way resembles French cooking or the Mediterranean diet. You will not be deprived of your favorite foods. Did you ever imagine that the French paradox could be due to the smaller portions French people eat, combined with lots of delicious juicy stews and some wine? By the way, no raw foods are required on the AGE-Less program. As you'll see in Parts 2 and 3, you will reap great benefits, even if you do not cut calories. The AGE-Less Way is not just a weight-reduction regimen and is, therefore, not a diet in the conventional sense.

For instance, some of us may be required to remain on a high-calorie diet, for different health reasons, which invariably complicates the situation. If you are in this category, simply trimming your AGE consumption, by changing the way food is prepared, but not calories, will drop down your AGEs to a level that your body can safely handle. This change will give you all the benefits of a reduced oxidant load while still enjoying tasty foods. No matter what your starting point is, with time you will get to where you need to be.

In Part 3 of this book, you will find simple but creative recipes, daily menus, and lots of tips on how to reduce the amount of AGEs in your diet while preserving and savoring the taste of your food. There will be plenty of information to help ease your transition to an AGE-Less lifestyle, since it does not require a change in either the amount or type of food you eat.

Case Study #1: Maureen E.

Age: 58
BEFORE: 142 lbs; BMI 23; 1500-1700 calories/day; 17,000 kU AGE/day
AFTER: 135 lbs; BMI 22; 1500-1700 calories/day; 8,000 kU AGE/day

RESULTS: Lost 7 lbs; reduced BMI by one point; reduced plasma glucose from 130 mg/dl to 98 mg/dl; reduced plasma insulin from 20 ng/dl to 9 ng/dl; reduced level of inflammatory marker CRP by 65%

Maureen E. is a fifty-eight-year-old physical therapy and exercise physiology expert and an ex-tap dancer who loves fresh, non-processed foods. She never had a problem with weight and exercised regularly. Nonetheless, when she developed a medical problem, she was forced to bed rest or no vigorous activity for about five months. A large congenital cyst was discovered in her lower back that had to be surgically removed. It became infected, and this forced her to undergo more surgery and prolonged postsurgical care. During that time she gained twenty pounds (usually she weighed around 125 pounds), and felt tired and without energy for the first time in her life, which shocked her.

She was told that she had "mild" diabetes and was instructed to go on a diet. But Maureen became frustrated because she had always eaten healthfully and worked physically hard all day. She became quite hungry when she cut her diet back to less than 1500 kcal/day. For a person who walked on foot everywhere, she now had trouble standing and sitting, and even her sleep was interrupted often.

So she decided to try the AGE-Less Way. We had her bring her calorie level back up to 1500-1700 calories a day and resume eating the foods she loved, but instructed her on how to prepare them the AGE-Less Way. She ate non-toasted bread, oatmeal, or boiled eggs for breakfast; meatloaf or chicken stews with rice and beans, lots of salads and fresh vegetables for dinner. Maureen loved to help with the neighborhood's weekly fresh veggies and fruit shopping from wholesale markets, which allowed all of them to economically purchase organic foods.

Two weeks after she started the AGE-Less Way, she found that she had begun to lose weight and felt more like herself. Both her blood glucose and insulin had improved almost to the normal range. She noticed she slept better. She returned to her normal level of daytime activity and in four weeks she had lost a total of eight pounds. At her normal weight, she was talking about dancing again and generally felt peppier.

"I would like to pass what I learned along to all my clients," she said. "Other diets might have been good for many overweight persons, but not for me. Calories were not my real problem. With the AGE-Less Way, my extra weight came off quite fast without losing muscle strength. I use my muscles a lot in my line of work. The biggest almost magical difference with AGE-Less food for me was that I got this feeling of normalcy almost immediately. And, you never have to go hungry or miss out on much. AGE-Less foods to me do not seem very different."

Chapter 4:
The Trojan Horse of Disease

The New Epidemics

Let's now take another step forward to look at food and disease. We know that AGEs are a normal part of our metabolism. Due to our American diet, too many AGEs enter our body with food. Hidden in plain sight, AGEs deplete our defenses long before we have a clue. This can leave us less protected against disease.

For instance, diabetes, and heart disease top every list of major health risks. These diseases have become so common as to have been officially designated as epidemics. This should ring an alarm, if not cause panic. The term *epidemic* was previously reserved for only those lethal infectious diseases that would periodically sweep across the world and wipe out millions of people and their livestock, like the bubonic plague or the Spanish flu. Thanks to medical and public health advances, these epidemics have now become rare in the Western world.

However, the calm did not last long. New epidemics of a different kind emerged, which posed a less immediate threat to life, but just as lethal. Diabetes, and heart and kidney diseases are the most common. Obesity is seemingly omnipresent, but it has not been called a disease yet. These epidemics are almost all related to nutrition and food, not to infectious diseases and, amazingly, not only to bad genes.

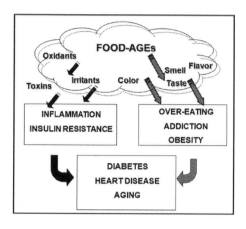

Figure 4: Most foods today are industrially modified and heat-treated. They are rich in colorful and flavorful AGEs, that increase appetite and drive over-eating and body weight gain. Not everyone becomes obese. But most people eat too many AGEs. AGEs can cause Inflammation and Insulin Resistance. Both lead to disease, like diabetes, heart disease and faster aging.

We now know that AGEs are elevated in all of these conditions. In this chapter we take a brief look at AGEs as a potential cause for diabetes, pre-diabetes, heart and kidney disease and how they can act as a connecting thread between our current food environment and them (**Figure 4**). Later, we will learn how the AGE-Less Way can break up this link as it strengthens our core health.

Setting the Stage

Diabetes is among the most common chronic diseases of the developed world. According to the American Diabetes Association, there are more than thirty million diabetics in the United States today, and an additional forty to sixty million people with pre-diabetes heading in that direction. There are more than five million people who do not even know they have diabetes and the number of newly diagnosed cases of diabetes is expected to double every ten years in the United States. Diabetes is now the leading cause of cardiovascular and kidney disease.

Diabetes develops when the body either does not make enough insulin (Type 1 Diabetes) or when the functions of insulin are blocked from allowing glucose to enter the cells (Type 2 Diabetes). Insulin is the hormone needed to bring sugar inside our cells and use it as energy. If insulin levels are too low or our cells do not respond to it in a normal way (that is they are somehow blocked from using insulin), the levels of the unused glucose would rise outside the cells and be detected in the blood. In an attempt to overcome the block, more insulin would be produced by the pancreatic islets. This situation may continue for years, or until the pancreas can no longer produce insulin and blood glucose rises even further. This type of diabetes (Type 2 Diabetes) is the most common form among adults.

Pre-Diabetes

Too much fat in the body makes our cells less responsive to insulin. This problem, called "insulin resistance", can be a huge problem because it is insulin that makes it possible for cells to take in glucose and convert it into energy. It is like not being able to take air into our lungs. Insulin levels in our blood rise as the body tries to use it to push glucose into cells, putting strain on the pancreatic islets. More fat leads to even higher levels of both insulin and glucose, as they both circle aimlessly outside the cells. Meanwhile, tissues are practically starving, since little or no glucose comes in to provide energy. Strange as it seems, the more we eat, and the fatter we get, the more our cells starve. Often this ends up in true diabetes, as the islets get fatigued, stop producing insulin altogether, and blood sugar rises to excessive levels. Insulin resistance, however, can also go on for many years quietly before diabetes completely develops.

Since this condition is related to over-nutrition, often with signs of "bad" cholesterol, high blood pressure, and heart problems, it is called the metabolic syndrome. This syndrome affects 25% to 40% of adults in the United States. This is a staggering reality, since it frequently ends up in Type 2 Diabetes. Since it causes no obvious symptoms, it often remains unrecognized. This is one of the reasons that the metabolic syndrome is so prevalent in the United States and Europe, and is spreading to the rest of the world. Unfortunately, people do not go to the doctor just because they are overweight.

Why be concerned? For one, while bad signs can be quiet for some time, they can suddenly tip the balance and turn toward diabetes, heart disease or high blood pressure, and even premature death. In countless instances where people unexpectedly suffered a heart attack or a stroke, it turns out that there were clear signs of trouble all along but went unrecognized. It was the rule for the metabolic syndrome to affect older adults. Now it is very common among younger persons, even adolescents.

The Chicken or the Egg

Until very recently, it was believed that AGEs were mostly products of our own sugars and they were only dangerously elevated when our sugar was high, as in uncontrolled diabetes. This is no longer true, as we have seen. So, which is the "chicken" and which is the "egg": AGEs or sugar? AGEs are a normal part of our metabolism. They are always present, as is oxygen, glucose, and free radicals. It is when AGE levels become excessive that they are toxic. The AGE-diabetes connection is all about excess. An overload of AGEs, coupled with high blood glucose levels, poses a serious health threat.

We have already seen the close relationship between food AGEs, blood AGEs and blood insulin, even in persons without diabetes. High levels of AGEs are associated with high insulin levels. This is a very important connection, since increased insulin is a sign of insulin resistance, the metabolic syndrome, and diabetes. Also, high AGEs are tied to *bad* cholesterol (high levels of low density lipoprotein, LDL), a combination that can make healthy persons more vulnerable to diabetes. The *good* cholesterol, HDL, tends to follow the reverse pattern, the higher the AGEs, the lower the HDL. This is also alarming since too low HDL levels are a risk for heart disease.

What then about persons who already have diabetes? They have at least twice as many AGEs in their blood than healthy persons. This was the case, even if their blood glucose was carefully controlled (hemoglobin A1c in the normal range). Those with high AGEs also had higher inflammation. In other words, AGEs were too high, no matter how well they tried to regulate their blood glucose levels. This could be where our thinking went wrong before: keeping the sugar down does not necessarily keep AGEs in check.

Before long, we figured out that there was much we had missed and much that could be gained from the AGE-Less Way for diabetic patients, just as it was for non-diabetics. The proof as always was in the pudding. A group of our diabetic volunteers was offered an AGE-Less Way plan, that is, a diet with the necessary calories (1,500-2000 kcal/day), but with about half the amount of AGEs (about 8000 kU/day, instead of 15,000 kU/day) for about six weeks. There was no change in any of their anti-diabetes medicines. The first clues were quite exciting. There was a noticeable effect not only on blood AGEs, which went down by about one third, but also on the overall inflammatory state. Within a mere few weeks, the AGE-Less Way had interrupted the vicious cycle of high AGEs and inflammation in a way that years of medical treatment had failed to achieve. The concept was simple and consistent with what we had already learned.

Confirmation of our suspicions came however with yet another study in Type 2 Diabetic patients who, despite multiple drugs, still had too high plasma insulin levels. Most were overweight and had elevated LDL and triglycerides (bad lipids), or low HDL (good) and, as expected, high AGEs. By the end of the two- to three-month exposure to an AGE-Less Way program, circulating blood AGEs fell by one half (from around 16 U/ml to the normal range, 8-10 U/ml). Most surprisingly, there was a striking decrease in plasma insulin levels (by 40%). This meant that patients on the AGE-Less Way became much less insulin resistant and their over-worked pancreas was no longer under the same stress. In other words, the AGE-Less Way made diabetes easier to control. If this was to be maintained over time, it might even improve diabetes and prevent heart and kidney complications. It might even reverse the condition itself.

This was despite the fact that particular attention had to be paid to ensure that there was no lowering of calories, fat, or other nutrients in these patients. With these facts in mind, it is likely that the AGE-Less diet facilitated the metabolism of stored fat in some subjects. Evidently, this was helped by an improvement in how the body utilizes its own insulin and glucose, a striking result not achieved by the multiple medications they were taking. Moreover, these clinical results perfectly matched the findings from our animal models.

There was also a clear loss in body weight in some overweight patients (by ~7-10 pounds) over a period of just four months. A number of them reported, not without a certain glee, that they shed pounds easier while on the AGE-Less Way than on other regimens.

Case Study #2: Michele T.

Age: 36

BEFORE: 140 lbs; BMI 25; 1500 calories/day; 14,000 kU AGEs/day; A1c 8.1%; fasting glucose 110 mg/dl; LDL-cholesterol 124 mg/dl

AFTER: 133 lbs; 1500 calories/day; 7,000 kU AGEs/day; A1c 6.5%; fasting glucose 80 mg/dl; LDL-cholesterol 98 mg/dl

RESULTS: Lost 7 lbs; reduced A1c level by about 2 percentage points; lowered LDL and fasting glucose

Michele has had Type 1 Diabetes since age nine. She always kept detailed records on her blood glucose and food intake and reviewed them with her physician. Even though she followed a very measured diet and exercise program and took insulin several times a day, she often felt tired, easily gained weight, and had extreme difficulty keeping her blood glucose under control.

She felt that she had to give up opportunities to go out for dinner, since she could not figure out how to prevent glucose from getting out of control. After she married, her husband depended on her for cooking, which she loved to do, but because he liked wonderful breads, steaks, chips and cakes —the things she should not have—she slowly found herself unable to stay away from all that. She put on weight gradually and more during her pregnancy. After giving birth to her daughter, she found it difficult to lose the extra weight, even though she tried hard and added exercise a couple of times a week for the next two years. She saw no change. All the demands of her health interfered with her personal life and she began to feel depressed.

Our first interview revealed a young woman with an intelligent and bright personality. Her diabetes was not well controlled. Her HbA1c was 8.1% (3 points above the normal value). Her blood glucose was 110 mg/dl. She knew she had put on extra weight, but she did not have any of the usual diabetic complications, except for protein in urine, which meant that she could soon develop kidney or vascular disease. She mainly broiled or pan-fried meat every day, mostly chicken, fish, and sometimes pork. In addition, she often had to resort to high sugar and calorie snacks to avoid or recover from low blood sugar due to over-shooting with insulin.

After two months on the AGE-Less Way, her weight dropped by seven pounds, to 133 pounds, her blood glucose was normal, HbA1c was 6.5 % (down by 2 points) and her circulating LDL-cholesterol was also lower (from 124 to 98 mg/dl). Her serum AGE levels and inflammatory markers were decreased by 40%, CRP was down by 70%, TNF alpha down by 30% and plasma 8-isoprostanes (lipid oxidants) down by 55%. Another significant fact was that protein was no longer detectable in her urine.

She commented that it was the first time she did not find it difficult to control her blood sugar, felt more energetic, had less frequent ups and downs of her blood sugar and had a "much clearer head." She could take her personal "crises" and those of her young family in stride. While she was initially afraid of starting the AGE-Less Way, she now found that preparing AGE-Less meals was becoming infinitely easier and just as tasty as before for both herself and her family. She was motivated to learn about how AGEs worked, both on herself and those around her, including her parents. She also wondered why this has not been recommended for all persons with diabetes.

The Heart: Always the Center of Attention

The overall mortality due to cardiovascular disease (CVD) has decreased by about 30% in the United States, partially due to the availability of new drugs and changes in dietary habits. It is an encouraging fact that the intense campaigns to reduce smoking, eat healthier, and use drugs that lower cholesterol levels have reduced mortality from heart disease. Despite these gains, heart disease remains the most common cause of death in America today. More than 50% of all deaths in the adult population in this country are due to heart and blood vessel problems. Diabetes is one of the biggest causes of these same problems. Contrary to the expectations, several large scale clinical trials have failed to establish even such rudimentary facts as the usefulness of tight sugar control or of antioxidants in cardiovascular disease, the number one killer of persons with diabetes. These costly studies consumed millions of dollars and appear to have wasted decades of research.

> *There is a critical balance between* <u>genes</u> *that carry the potential for a disease, and* <u>triggers</u> *that actually bring out the disease. AGEs in the ordinary American diet qualify as such* <u>triggers.</u>

Cardiovascular disease frequently appears first in the form of hypertension (also known as high blood pressure) or as atherosclerosis (which is the hardening of the arteries). It is no secret that the heart is a pump. We depend on it to push blood from the heart to all the parts of the body. Blood vessels are basically distensible tubes that stretch to accommodate the blood pushed through them at a high pressure with each beat. Gradually, as we grow older, certain changes take place. At first there is a slight stiffness of the normally supple and elastic walls. When the arteries become rigid, they do not stretch enough with each heartbeat. This means that the pressure inside the vessel increases. The only way arteries can handle the higher pressure is to build thicker and stronger walls. As you can imagine, the thickened blood vessels also have a smaller opening, which reduces the flow of blood to the organs. Signals are then sent to the heart to pump harder, which can lead to high blood pressure. This forces the heart to become enlarged and have thicker and more muscular walls. Eventually, the heart becomes unable to pump blood well. This vicious cycle leads to a condition called heart failure. Stiffening of the heart is a gradual process that occurs long before it is diagnosed and often in early adult life.

Table 4-3: How AGEs Cause Heart Disease
and Hardening of Arteries

- They stick to heart and arterial walls, trap cholesterol and form "rusty" deposits, causing inflammation and harm.

- Cause vessels to become leaky.

- Build bridges that tie-up connective tissue collagen making vessels rigid

- Mobilize immune cells, scavenger macrophages (pac-men) that can cause inflammation

- Cause blood clots to form, causing a heart attack or a stroke

---

What do AGEs have to do with all these changes? Almost everything: AGEs can either form inside or slip through the lining of the vessel wall. AGEs then attach to the collagen matrix and make the heart thicker and more rigid, or act as oxidants that irritate vascular tissues and cause inflammation. AGEs can also turn circulating lipids into a rust-like material that coats the inside of the blood vessels, gradually closing down the lumen. Blood vessels can become so clogged that they no longer let blood pass through.

The immune system responds to all these annoying events by sending macrophages into the vascular wall to clean up AGEs. Macrophages gobble up everything in sight. The problem begins when they over-ingest AGEs, causing them to sputter potent inflammatory substances, harmful to the very tissues they came out to protect. They can irritate platelets (tiny cells that control bleeding), tweaking them to produce dangerous clots that can suddenly block the blood flow in an already narrow vessel and lead to a heart attack or a stroke. Heart attacks can also be caused by "fatty-rusty" plugs made up of AGE-cholesterol.

Many studies were necessary to nail down these events and put them together as in a giant puzzle. In one such study, we worked with animals that have a genetic tendency to produce too much bad cholesterol, causing them heart attacks and death at an early age. Remarkably, when given the AGE-Less diet, these mice lived without heart attacks, even if they got diabetes. There is a critical interplay between *genes* that hold the potential of a disease, and *triggers* that actually bring out the disease. One message of these studies is that AGEs in the ordinary American diet qualify as such *triggers*. More importantly, the simple avoidance of the AGE-triggers can drastically change the odds for developing a life-threatening disease, despite a strong genetic predisposition. In a nutshell, if you avoid the trigger - all you have to do is sit on your hands! - then you could avoid the disease.

Human Experience

Naturally the next question was whether this applies to humans. Two simple experiments said "yes" to this question; one done with the help of healthy adults and the other done in patients with diabetes. The first involved simply drinking a concentrate of a sugar-free dark soda, in this case diet cola, which contained about 10,000 kU of AGEs in a normal sized glass. Volunteers that drank this cola showed abnormal blood flow to the arm during a special test, which indicated a sudden malfunction of the arteries in response to the cola, followed –and confirmed - by a spike in certain markers of vascular injury in the blood. This amounted to a new and important observation because consumption of dark drinks (AGE-laden) could now be tied to vascular disease using the same link, AGEs. As we learned, the caramel content of these dark drinks is a source of AGEs, which promotes arterial changes that - if consumed regularly and in the excessive amounts typically seen today - could lead to cardiovascular disease.

Changes in blood flow and markers of vascular injury can be even more worrisome for persons with diabetes because of their propensity for vascular disease. Our second experiment was carried out in two groups of patients with Type 2 Diabetes. Both groups were provided a solid food meal with identical calories. However, one group received a meal cooked by AGE-Less Way methods – and had a low AGE content –, while the other received a meal prepared by regular methods (AGE-rich). The results were similar to the experiment done with healthy people as described above: above on vascular blood flow, as indicators of vascular injury in blood intensified, but only in diabetics who consumed the regular (AGE-rich) meal. This lead to the same conclusion: too many AGEs are oxidants that can cause disease. By flooding and overwhelming our natural defenses, they can weaken vascular function. This is especially true in the presence of diabetes.

Whether healthy or with diabetes, our arteries are vulnerable to offending substances. These include not only excess salt, sugar and fat, but also food AGEs. There is now good clinical evidence that many and repeated small "shocks" to the system can lead to the development or worsening of cardiovascular disease. There was a clear warning implicit in these findings, especially for those who already have a heart condition.

One may well wonder whether, in the absence of apparent symptoms, there are true long-term benefits to be expected by following an AGE-Less Way. While larger and longer clinical studies will be addressing these questions, the signs are all positive: the virtual plummeting to normal levels of AGEs, of inflammation and of vascular markers. These all promise that the end result will certainly be worthwhile when we consider the surreptitious nature of heart disease and diabetes. There is no doubt that we stand to gain many long-term health benefits.

Case Study #3: X

Age: 78
BEFORE: 175 lbs; BMI 30; 2100 calories/day; 18,000 kU AGEs/day; blood pressure 165/105 mmHg; LDL cholesterol 248 mg/dl; HDL cholesterol 42 mg/dl
AFTER: 168 lbs; BMI 28.4; 2030 calories/day; 10,000 kU AGEs/day; blood pressure 150/90 mmHg; LDL cholesterol 215 mg/dl; HDL cholesterol 64 mg/dl
RESULTS: Lost 7 lbs; reduced CRP inflammation by 60%

Diana is a novelist and a university professor of English writing. Being of Italian descent, she loves to cook Italian food and throw great parties with the finest Italian pasta dishes. She knew every store and bakery in the city and made sure that her ingredients were "original." She did not do physical exercise, per se, but took long walks with her husband. Her favorite hobby was talking up a storm with fellow writers and other artists as she cooked and served delicious food. Fifteen years ago, she had a small stroke, which fortunately resolved completely. In addition to medications for her "cholesterol, and mild heart condition," she was also put on a low fat diet. She began swimming lessons and liked it. Much to her dismay, her weight did not change much.

On interview, her intake of AGEs was a hefty 18,000 kU/day, mostly due to her love of Italian sausages and cheeses. She ate sufficient amounts of fish, olive oil, and vegetables. Diana's problems were that she fatigued easily and was unable to go up and down the stairs as easily as she once could; one floor was enough for her to be out of breath. Her gait had become particularly syncopated; she would take very short steps and get dizzy often. She was told that she had hardened arteries and this probably affected the blood supply to the nerves in her feet. However, she was not told of diabetes.

Diana's lifestyle is not easy to categorize as unhealthy. In fact, it was not too different from a Mediterranean diet. Diana cooked Italian but in the American way, that is, with too much high heat and broiling or frying the meat. She would often fry cheese. New studies have now shown that even a Mediterranean diet must be prepared in the AGE-Less Way if it is to maintain its beneficial effects. Since Diana was an intelligent and motivated woman, it was not difficult to imagine that she would see the value of the AGE-Less Way. In fact, she came up with a number of interesting ideas about how to reinvent traditional Italian cooking! Within the span of two months, her high bad cholesterol (LDL) level was noticeably less, and her good HDL-cholesterol increased. Her blood pressure was, for the first time, closer to her physician's target. She had signed up for physical therapy that helped gain strength in her legs and control her balance. What was most important for her was the realization that she could continue to eat what she wanted, without cutting out much else other than sausage, cold-cuts and cheeses. She could still have lean meat, plenty of fish and cheese—she loved low-fat mozzarella—as long as she used low-temperature heat in her kitchen, shorter periods of cooking, and plenty of water, spices, and herbs. She used olive oil quite often but was reminded that even this type of oil could have as much AGEs as any other if it was not very fresh (difficult to know) or if it was used in cooking or frying. She loved fruits and salads, as well as fresh Italian bread, which she ate instead of toasted Italian bread or cereals that contain lots of fructose. She replaced Italian cakes that often have butter and high-fat cream with poached pears and apples in Italian wine sauce.

The Kidneys: The Silent Heroes

While everyone agrees that the heart is the eternal symbol of life and happiness, few view the kidneys in that romantic way. We are wrong on this count! The kidneys, each no bigger than a fist, shoulder several heavy-duty jobs, one of which is to protect the heart itself. Although truly heroic, they tend to be silent !Their best known function is the removal of toxic waste products from the blood in the form of urine. They also control the crucial balance between water and salt in the body. Kidneys play an important role in the hormones that regulate blood pressure, the production of red blood cells and bone growth. Such vital functions explain their high blood flow. They have an enormous reserve capacity; nearly one and a half of our kidneys can be removed and the remaining half a kidney can still cope with our day-to-day needs. Another important function, that is only now becoming recognized, is their role in expelling AGEs from the body.

The kidneys are extremely adaptive organs. But let's face it, there are limits. We calculated that the amount of AGEs pouring into the body with each meal exceeds the capacity of the kidney to remove them by at least two to three fold. Imagine all those non-cleared, toxic AGEs that end up back in our tissues each day, month, and year. This should give you an idea of the enormous burden of AGEs that we carry through life.

As with all organs, the kidneys accumulate AGEs over time. The process is similar to the hardening of the arteries, something like hardening of the kidneys, known as nephrosclerosis (from the Greek *nephron*, "kidney," and *sclerosis*, "hard"). This fairly common condition escapes detection because of the enormous reserve capacity of the kidneys. However, as kidney reserves are diminished, the ability to excrete AGEs and other oxidants decreases. This causes even more AGEs to be stashed in tissues, including the kidneys themselves. In short, because kidneys are constantly exposed to the entire blood volume, they bear the brunt of damage due to excess AGEs.

Blood AGEs constantly flood the kidneys and eventually cause enough oxidant damage that reduces the kidneys' ability to get rid of waste products, and control water and salt. Injury to the kidney reduces their ability to preserve precious proteins, for instance albumin, leading to its presence in the urine. The presence of albumin in the urine (albuminuria) also signals a reduced ability to regulate oxidants, i.e., AGEs. Since oxidants can damage vital organs, and it is the kidneys' job to control them, signs of kidney damage (like albuminuria) serve as early warnings that the heart, brain and other organs are at risk. Thanks to their enormous resilience and reserve, the kidneys can work well for a long time before problems are recognized. Since the signs of kidney disease are indirect, this may be detected by the "accidental" finding of albumin in the urine. Other hints include the presence of high blood pressure (hypertension), low blood count (anemia), or swelling of the legs (edema). However, even a small decrease in the kidneys' ability to detoxify AGEs, could mean heart and vascular problems down the road. Decreased kidney function often becomes recognized only after the onset of other serious problems, such as diabetes, high blood pressure, or stroke.

Now for the good news, which should not come as a surprise if you've read the previous chapters. It is clear that the AGE-Less Way can help preserve and may restore some aspects of kidney function. The kidneys can quickly recover at least one crucial function: their unique ability to excrete oxidants. How did we discover this? By conducting several clinical trials in both diabetic and non-diabetic subjects with different types and degrees of kidney disease. After only four weeks on the AGE-Less Way program, the amount of AGEs excreted in the urine nearly doubled, showing that this critical aspect of kidney function was restored.

All discussion on the kidneys these days starts with the diabetic kidney, since diabetes is the most common cause for kidney failure. Abnormal kidney function is evident in a large number -30 to 40% - of diabetic persons, but only a handful of "bad" genes have been incriminated. So the fear of kidney disease looms over every person with diabetes and severely affects their lives. It is well known that high blood sugar causes damage to the kidney and that maintaining a normal blood sugar level helps slow this process down. Since keeping the kidneys healthy protects the health of many other organs, patients with diabetes take special precautions to avoid kidney injury. Balancing blood glucose minute-to-minute and within a narrow range places enormous pressure on patients and their families. And there is still little in the way of protection for this disease. Despite decades of research, we are not much closer to the answer.

There is reason to believe that increased AGEs due to high glucose are partly the cause of kidney trouble in diabetes. Countless studies, our own included, have shown that AGEs indeed damage the kidneys. The most convincing evidence is based on the fact that blocking the formation of AGEs by special anti-AGE drugs protects the kidneys from the effects of diabetes in animals. Some of these studies were conducted in our laboratory, while others are at the stage of clinical trials or on their way to becoming available for clinical use.

Recent findings, however, deserve close attention. Food AGEs seem to be at least as important for diabetic kidneys as is high blood sugar. We tested this theory in diabetic mice that happened to also be genetically susceptible to kidney disease. We replaced their standard mouse chow (which is rich in AGEs) with an AGE-Less chow that had only half the amount of AGEs. In just a few months, it was clear that the AGE-Less diet had almost completely protected these diabetic mice from kidney disease.

Two points are worth noting here. First, the diet was effective despite a persistently elevated blood sugar. Second, despite defective genes, kidney disease did not develop. Remember? No trigger, no trouble. Diabetic kidney disease may have less to do with high sugar and a great deal more with high AGEs, most of them from food.

The practical message was that lower consumption of AGE-rich foods is simple and effective, and it can provide protection against this devastating complication.

A Worthy Cause

Experts believe that after about age forty kidney function declines. Based on a large cross-sectional study, decreased kidney function was found in one third of all older Americans, a number that keeps climbing up. Since the kidneys affect such a large array of vital organs, this raises great concern. The cause for this decline in renal function is unknown. Could it be somehow linked to the general inflammation of older age and, if so, what is its origin?

To address this question, we injected pre-made AGEs into young healthy laboratory mice and found that they soon developed kidney changes resembling diabetic or old kidneys. If they were given AGE-inhibitors, however, this did not happen. A similar protection was noted in old mice that were fed an AGE-Less diet. The conclusion was that food AGEs over time can cripple kidney function, even without diabetes, and that a lower consumption of AGEs keeps kidneys healthy, as well as a more youthful heart. No wonder that these mice lived longer and healthier lives.

The evident question was once again, what about us humans? Older patients with kidney disease have AGE levels seven to ten times above the normal level. We learned that the major reason for this is that the food AGE intake far surpasses the kidneys' excretion rate.

In one study, half of our participants were instructed how to maintain an AGE-Less Way program at home, that is to avoid excessive dry heat during cooking. Their AGE intake was set to about half the usual amount, but the diet was nutritionally complete. After just one month, much to their surprise, blood AGE levels decreased by more than 50%. There was a similar decrease in markers of inflammation within this short interval. These results were remarkable, since the participants of this study had long standing kidney disease, known for its resistance to treatment. The study was much too short to expect a change in measures of kidney function, such as serum creatinine or albumin in the urine. But we should not ignore the fact that the kidneys doubled their ability to clear toxic AGEs from the blood and put them into the urine, a fact that was in part responsible for the reduction of inflammation in these people. Efficient elimination of AGEs continued as long as the patients remained on the AGE-Less diet, but if they reverted to their old habits, the benefits were soon lost. An obvious message here is that, because kidney disease is difficult to reverse, there is a sure benefit in staying away from AGE-laden foods and do it as a way of keeping your kidneys rejuvenated and your life safer.

The AGE-Less Way may be the easiest way to avoid kidney trouble and stay healthy. In the long run it is a very worth-while investment.

Case Study #4: Mary X.

Age: 58

BEFORE: 172 lbs; BMI 28; 16,000 kU AGEs/day; 1600 kcal/day; blood pressure 168/110 mmHg

AFTER: 164 lbs; BMI 26.7; 7,000-8,000 kU AGEs/day; 1700 kcal/day; blood pressure 146/95 mmHg

RESULTS: Lost 8 lbs; reduced CRP inflammation by 58%; lowered blood pressure dramatically

Mary complained about chronic fatigue, pains in her back and legs, and difficulty of getting up in the morning. She has a family history of kidney disease, but Mary had no problems until five years ago. She has been treated for high blood pressure, but has not managed to get it down enough. She used to swim or play tennis almost daily , but now she exercised only once or twice a week. She was preparing meals almost always by broiling and frying, which is what her husband and children preferred. She loved to cook and eat out. She was careful about salt while cooking, but she had never heard about how to prepare meals by using less heat. Although Mary was trying hard to reduce the intake of calories, she was still overweight and could not control her blood pressure. She tried to avoid sweetened drinks, but drank more than four diet colas a day. Mary is on two medications for her blood pressure.

According to Mary, her most important problem was her kidney disease, and the second was her blood pressure. The third was her excessive weight—not so much for the appearance, she clarified, but because it made her tired, and she realized it affected her body from tip to toe. For Mary, the most important issue was to get her energy back so that she would be able to take long walks with her husband and kids.

When we evaluated her meal preparation methods one month after starting on the AGE-Less Way, we found that she had managed extremely well to keep meals as nutritious and as tasty as before. The AGE content was lowered by about one-half to two-thirds.

Within the first few weeks, Mary reported that she could now adapt all family meals to the AGE-Less Way, and no one in her family complained of a difference. After two months, Mary reported that she had a sense of well-being that she had not felt in years and her energy and optimism had returned. She had lost about eight pounds. She knew that the true benefit was mostly working inside her body. We explained to her that her AGEs were almost to the levels of a person without kidney problems and that her inflammatory markers had plummeted. She liked to say that now she had found a way to "put some savings away," referring to restored anti-oxidant defenses. This helped her to regain much-needed strength to fight her kidney disease. She loved to talk about how her new diet was still rich in vegetables and fruits and, even though it included meat, this was now AGE-Less meat. Her family eventually expressed to her that they had noticed the changes from fried foods and grilled steaks to stews, soups and steamed dishes, and that they loved these new meals.

Mary X. is someone who values taking control of her life. This was reflected in how she felt about herself at the last meeting . She immediately shared her story with those around her. She had learned quickly and well.

Chapter 5:
Aging and AGE

Human Age in History

When it comes down to health, despite all the open questions and problems that remain to be solved, one thing is certain: in our part of the world, we live for many more years now than at any other time in human history. Forcing the limits of nature has got to be one of the greatest feats of modern science.

Yet, we would give a lot to hold onto our strength, mobility, and mental faculties, and to push back disease and debility for as long as possible. On this score, we have reasons to be skeptical. The results of countless "fountains of youth" remain modest; many have unpleasant or harmful side effects, cost a fortune, or just don't work. All the while, the diseases of late life continue to flourish and spread.

So, if a longer life span does not equal a longer health span, what do we need it for? How can we reap the fruits of this promise? Human health has evolved over millions of years, and over this vast period of time life span changed at an uneven pace. Until the last millennium, the life span of *Homo sapiens*, our ancestor, averaged at only about forty years, just twice that of the ape. It took tens of thousands of years for our life span to double again.

This change in life span was hugely influenced by demographic shifts. One such shift was the transition from a low-fat plant-based diet to an omnivorous modern style with a diet high in animal fat and protein. With the industrial revolution, life gave way to an environment that favored longer survival. However, life-threatening infections continued, even in agrarian societies. Scholars have observed that, in terms of lifespan, such patterns may have forced the natural selection of those groups that adapted to a more energy efficient pattern of feeding. Higher fat intake allowed these groups to store energy for periods of famine, and their immune systems were better prepared to successfully fight off infections. This led to societies that created systems for efficient food production and better public health. In other words, until about two centuries ago, it was natural selection that dictated how long humans lived. Science and technology then took over the reins and in just a short period of time, brought about a huge expansion of human longevity. This gave a new meaning to getting old.

What is it then that causes us to age today, and is there anything to help us "age well," since it cannot be skipped altogether? A few definitions may be useful. Among the most cited causes of aging today are: too much oxidant stress, free radicals, diminished anti-oxidants, and inflammation. Normal cellular events depend on small amounts of very reactive free radicals. If in excess, however, these radicals can cause "bystander" oxidant damage. What causes this excess of free radicals to be generated in the first place? There are different views and endless debates on this issue. But here is a clue that should sound familiar: free radicals are standard byproducts of those same chemical reactions that create our familiar AGEs.

A Trade-off for Years

It is worthwhile to introduce at this point some of the important effects that food and nutrients can have on aging. Over the last fifty years or more, many studies tried to sort out whether specific nutrients or just excessive calories can cause disease or affect the speed of aging. The results have been quite variable, with one exception: across a wide spectrum of animal species, the effects of aging were unequivocally delayed by drastically reducing total calorie consumption (40-60%), leading to a considerably longer lifespan. The calorie restriction (CR), it turned out, lowers free radical production, decreases oxidant damage and prevents unwanted DNA changes, inflammation and its effects. It is not surprising that the incidence of many chronic diseases of aging would decrease as well.

Since CR is accomplished by reducing total food intake, it necessarily results in a lower AGE intake, with fewer AGEs ending up in the body. So which is it that carries these benefits: the fewer calories, the reduced AGEs consumed with the diet, or both? To answer this, mice were given one of two diets; both with exactly the same calories, but one had only half the amount of AGEs (AGE-Less diet). All of the mice eventually got old, but those fed the AGE-Less diet kept their youthful heart and kidneys, a greater level of physical activity, less body fat and less diabetes; reasons for which they lived a lot longer.

A direct conclusion from these studies was that simply lowering AGEs in the food (by just one-half) may be enough to arrest oxidant damage and inflammation expected with older age and lead not only to a longer lifespan but, more importantly, to a better health-span. Food AGEs then, not just calories, might be a key to both age-related diseases and aging itself.

But how can we be sure whether this trade-off of AGEs for healthful years would work for us humans? Even a less drastic calorie restriction seems to hold promise. The fact remains, however, that it still requires substantial restrictions in food intake and this raises doubts as to its utility, especially as one becomes older. New drugs that can imitate the effects of calorie restriction, like *resveratrol*, have been gaining in popularity for the obvious reasons, but the jury is still out on these. It should be noted that while no drugs come without side effects and considerable expense, the AGE-Less Way plan is completely safe and economical. It might be a matter of time before these issues are sorted out and a combination of drugs, calorie and AGE restriction can be designed for an even longer and healthier life.

Old age affects every part and function of the body. Since we've already visited some of the most common problems, let us briefly talk about some other conditions that touch almost everyone: memory loss, eyesight, and skin wrinkles.

Case Study #5: Thomas J.

Age: 43
BEFORE: 153 lbs; BMI 24; 1700 calories/day; 15,000 kU AGEs/day
AFTER: 147 lbs; BMI 23; 1700 calories/day; 8,000 kU AGEs/day
RESULTS: Lost 6 lbs

Thomas J. is a nutritional biologist who heard me give a talk on the AGE-Less Way. He read about our work and concluded that the idea was fascinating, but questioned its practicality. What he was particularly interested in finding out was if the AGE-Less Way program would work as well as a calorie restriction diet. In other words, would his body weight go down together with AGEs and levels of inflammation if he continued to eat the same amount and type of food, but only changed the way of preparing it? Would other changes happen in his metabolism (for example, blood sugar or insulin)?

There were no prior reported studies in normal humans. He asked his wife, a real gourmet cook, if she would help work out the simple principles of the AGE-Less Way: to use less heat, more water and lemon or vinegar marinades before cooking and so on. He knew very well that to lose weight one had to reduce calories below what one needed to spend for energy. Simple, and correct, of course.

This time, however, he and his wife agreed to keep the same calories while they lowered their AGE intake. This was what Thomas found most difficult to "digest." He called us after three to four months on the AGE-Less Way to announce that he and his wife were excited. He noticed that eating the AGE-Less Way had actually helped him to lose about six pounds. His wife, who was smaller, lost five pounds (they were both of normal weight to begin with, even a little on the thin side). They had no trouble getting used to this way of cooking.

The aspect that was most fascinating to Thomas was that he did not have to try very hard because he did not have to lower his caloric intake. What was even more fascinating for him was that the two markers of inflammation in his blood, C-reactive protein [CRP] and tumor necrosis factor alpha [TNFα], were also lowered, even below the levels that he had previously thought were just fine. His blood levels of AGEs also went down by about 50%. This was exactly what calorie restriction was supposed to do. However, with calorie restriction, perhaps his weight would have to have gone far below normal. At this amount of food restriction and weight, his hunger would have more than likely made him unhappy.

His glucose and insulin did not seem to change very much, but this is the result we antici-pated in a relatively young man in good general health. If Thomas continues to follow the AGE-Less Way, he may hold onto his excellent health for a long time and remain at his appropriate weight. If you are not overweight, simply maintaining the AGE-Less Way will work on your health while you sleep and while you eat! If you are overweight, the AGE-Less Way works best when combined with other dietary guidelines. It will help normalize your weight and, perhaps, prevent the development of pre-diabetes or heart problems.

Thomas and his wife had fun designing gourmet dishes with lots of herbs and spices, stews, and casseroles. They often preferred this over going to restaurants, especially because the AGE-Less Way saved them a lot of money.

The Brain: Our Fortress

Dementias

One of the worst fears is the loss of mental capabilities. Memory, ability to concentrate, being connected, and learning can all decline with age. These changes can happen suddenly with a stroke, which occurs when a blood vessel in the brain becomes blocked by a clot, or they can settle in over many years with the gradual erosion of the intellect. The latter is called dementia or cognitive decline. There are many kinds of dementia; some are attributed to hardening or narrowing of brain arteries; others are thought to be due to lack of vitamins or important micronutrients, trauma, or infections.

Until the twentieth century, about a third of persons over age eighty were likely to develop some form of dementia. This number now doubles every four to five years after age sixty.

This trend is not just due to the fact that people now live longer lives. Most types of cognitive decline have been linked to the same diseases that have surged in the last fifty to seventy years: diabetes, heart and kidney disease, and high blood pressure. What about this uncanny coincidence? For example, diabetics are more likely to develop Alzheimer's disease than those without diabetes. This is particularly true for diabetics who have poorly controlled glucose levels. Most affected persons are concentrated in the United States and Europe, where the rising frequency of heart disease and diabetes coincides with the industrial revolution and its aftermath.

Why this increase? Scientists have considered everything, from genetic causes, to a lack of vitamins, to a loss of natural anti-oxidants, to too much stress and new environmental toxins. They point to oxidants of some sort that once inside the brain cause inflammation. Most now agree on this one count: All forms of dementia are attributed to inflammation and oxidant stress. Dementia due to old age has been linked to excessive free radicals inside the brain cells, leading to oxidant damage and the ever-present inflammation. Does this sound familiar?

More than a hundred years ago, researchers noticed that brain cells accumulated a kind of yellow-brown pigment called lipofuscin, regarded as cellular debris. The same pigment was also found in other organs, such as the heart, eyes, and kidneys, and was identified as a mix of oxidized lipids and proteins generally thought to be inert waste material that piled up over time. Suddenly it was found to contain AGEs, which are everything but inert. It took awhile for scientists to re-discover that AGEs are found in many areas of the brain and that their levels increase with age, just as brain function slows down.

Alzheimer's Disease

One of the more worrisome forms of dementia is Alzheimer's disease. It has been the most terrifying form because it can start at a younger age and rapidly become severe. It is important to discuss Alzheimer's disease in some detail since this remains the most common type of dementia in the elderly.

Alzheimer's disease is a slowly progressing disorder characterized by loss of brain cells and by the emergence of AGE-filled plaque-like deposits in areas that command memory. A typical early symptom is difficulty in recalling specific events, but brain changes may begin long before any symptoms appear. Women seem to be more susceptible to Alzheimer's disease, and while a family history of this disease or certain genetic traits are recognized as risk factors, there is usually no apparent cause.

What is more intriguing is that Alzheimer's disease and other dementias are now linked with other chronic diseases, like diabetes, high blood pressure, and the metabolic syndrome! As in these diseases, inflammation arises, only this time in the brain. The cause and significance of this inflammation continues to be widely debated. But is there any evidence to support a relationship between AGEs and Alzheimer's disease?

The brain is an exceptionally well-protected area. But over the years AGEs can skip over the protective barrier that separates the brain from the rest of the body, or slip between and inside the brain cells. A good analogy would be that of a fortress with walls crumbling after a long siege.

Once behind the brain barrier, AGEs bond with brain components, such as amyloid-beta, a fragment of a starchy protein common in the brain and thought as potentially harmful. The formation of these bonds forces amyloid-beta to fold up, just like an accordion, resulting in small deposits of protein. The deposits spread, forming larger aggregates, called plaques. AGEs inside brain cells also prompt the formation of fibrillar tangles (think of them as a mass of tangled hair). These tangles, together with the plaques, are hallmarks of Alzheimer's disease and both are thought to be quite injurious to the human brain. There is convincing evidence that AGEs can instigate or accelerate these changes, since certain AGE inhibitors, such as *aminoguanidine*, can abolish them in laboratory animals.

What is far more exciting is a recent study in mice that demonstrated dramatic changes in the brain of old mice fed an AGE-rich diet, in sharply contrast to equally old mice fed AGE-Less food: Less than one-half of brain AGEs went hand-in-hand with minimal amyloid-beta deposits and inflammation in the brains our AGE-Less mice.This highlighted how harmful overt consumption of AGE-foods can be to brain. The effects of the AGE-Less diet were indeed a most exciting development with a huge potential for us humans.

AGEs and Stroke

Even without forming plaques and tangles, AGEs can accumulate over the years around the brain's blood vessels or inside the brain cells. It follows that, in either case, there would be a response evoked by the brain's immune system, followed by localized inflammation that would remain silent for long periods of time, until disease takes over. This scenario led us to wonder if the presence of AGEs worsens the brain damage wrought by a stroke. Working with laboratory animals, we determined that,

 ....the extent of brain damage from a stroke is larger and more serious when the brain has higher levels of AGEs.

This could mean that food AGEs gaining entry into the brain can undermine its odds for recovery from trouble. To establish these findings in humans could take several decades more. But, as you read below, there may be new light shone on this question too.

Memory Loss

To get a glimpse at the relationship of AGEs to some of the most delicate functions of the human brain such as memory, we studied a large group of healthy men and women over the age of seventy-five who were in fairly good general health and completely self-sufficient. We worked closely with specialists who examined cognitive function by using a long list of memory tests (including what is called the Mini Mental State Exam) and other clinical predictors of dementia.

The results were interesting from the start. Even though these elderly persons were healthy at the time, there was an inverse correlation between their mental function and blood levels of AGEs: the higher the AGEs, the worse the brain function. During a follow-up period of about five years, a more powerful observation was made: there was a striking relationship between blood AGEs and the rapid rate at which mental function had diminished over these years. These findings are particularly important precisely because the study included only healthy persons. In other words, the changes could not have been as easily detected as if these people had higher AGEs due to diabetes or heart disease. So, we may soon have a simple test that could alert us to the likelihood of dementia. On the other hand, these changes were independent of variables that are important in dementia, such as age, gender or education. Thus far, these findings are the strongest available epidemiologic evidence that AGEs are toxic for the human brain. But they are all the more interesting since we now know that most of us consume an excess of AGEs with food and that we can reduce them easily and efficiently.

These findings also make good sense once tied to the previous chapters, on diabetes, heart or kidney disease. It is not difficult to figure out that if AGEs are present in the brain, they will cause inflammation and more rapid brain aging. Nor is it far-fetched to imagine AGEs as a common denominator between dementia and these conditions, nor that they can predispose us to mental decline. An important fact gleaned from this study was that levels of AGEs in the blood could probably help predict the earliest signs of brain dysfunction, or memory loss. Since we can now measure AGEs in the blood, there may be no need to look too far inside the brain to make an early diagnosis of impending dementia.

Assessing levels of blood AGEs in older adults and in the diet on a routine basis might make it possible to anticipate dementia or Alzheimer's disease, as with other chronic diseases. Since high levels of AGEs are toxic to the brain, opting for an AGE-Less Way of life could indeed help delay or avoid this devastating disease.

Who, in their right mind, could ignore such a bargain?

Sharp Focus and Clear Sight

The passing of years and a weakened health affect vision, the most precious of senses in many ways. An easy way to visualize how intricately related our age is to AGEs – aside from the experiment with the glass vial that contained sugar and egg-white discussed in Chapter 1 – is by telling the story of our lenses. The lenses in our eyes allow light to reach the retina so we can see. Lenses are made of translucent proteins, which allow the light to pass through without diffraction (or bending of the light waves) so we can enjoy perfectly clear vision. The lenses of children and young people are clear, like drops of pure water or crystal. In fact, the proteins inside them are named crystallins. The lenses of older adults become progressively opaque with age. This is often described as a "curtain of white water falling in front of one's eyes"—hence the Greek name *cataracts*. The lens is elastic and its shape can adjust to sharpen the focus on close up or far away objects. But with increasing age the lens gradually becomes inelastic. This is one reason that we lose the ability to focus and require new glasses. When the lens proteins are modified by AGEs they become yellowish and then brown, preventing the passage of light and ultimately blocking vision (**Figure 5**).

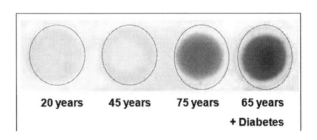

20 years   45 years   75 years   65 years
                                    + Diabetes

Figure 5: Cataracts or cloudy lenses, a common problem in aging or diabetes, are in large part due to AGEs. The darker color of AGEs (on the right) is easy to see in lenses removed from older or diabetic persons, but these changes had already started long before. A similar process unfolds in our vessels, heart, kidneys, brain. Only, there is no easy way for us to see it.

All this trouble begins when AGEs form on crystallins and build bridges between individual crystallin molecules. The AGEs disrupt the crystal-like organization of these proteins, and eventually form the solid dark brown mass called a cataract. What is the evidence that AGEs are involved? Cataracts are far more common whenever AGE levels are high, such as in diabetes and aging. When young laboratory mice were given AGEs, they developed cataracts identical to those of older animals. However, if the mice also received an AGE inhibitor, they did not develop cataracts. We now surgically replace damaged lenses with relative ease using synthetic lenses, but these can cause other problems, notably to other parts of the eye that cannot be repaired so easily.

Isn't it then infinitely safer to avoid risky procedures to our eyes, if this simply means learning early on to avoid food AGEs? Not long ago, people took care of their teeth by avoiding too many sweets or putting fluoride in the water - that is by taking simple preventive measures. This simple act of prevention is just the kind of pro-active thinking we need here. The AGE-less Way offers a sure way to keep our vision crystal clear and possibly safe from worse eye problems.

Let's Face It: Smooth Skin Goes a Long Way

The skin is the most noticeable mirror of poor health and old age. That is not surprising, since first and foremost it is in direct contact with the environment. Just being exposed to sun, air, and all kinds of pollutants make skin vulnerable to irritation, trauma, disease, and exhaustion.

It is a known fact that most common skin problems are due to inflammation, often referred to as dermatitis. Sunburn, a good example, is caused by ultraviolet light that causes skin cells to produce free radicals, which cause our familiar oxidant damage. An acute sunburn makes the skin red and painful (called erythema), but even low amounts of sun exposure on a repeated basis and the attendant oxidative damage can make skin wrinkled and inelastic.

Over time, AGEs too can have the similiar effects on skin. AGEs accumulate on proteins that do not get replaced very often, such as collagen. As AGEs build cross-bridges between collagen molecules, they make skin rigid and less elastic. Loss of elasticity and thickening leads to premature wrinkling and sagging.

The entire body is in a constant state of repair. Since our cells, including those of the skin, are constantly being replaced by new ones, the skin is a perfect example of this constant and extraordinary renewal process. The less the AGE burden, the smoother the turnover and up-keep, the better the healing and repair of normal skin. The less oxidant damage, the less the inflammation and the more youthful the skin remains over time.

Although skin is capable of repairing itself, an excess of AGEs can affect it in many ways. For example, skin cells can be irritated by AGEs and can respond by proliferating, making more skin than is needed, as if to shield us from harm. Some skin cells that are part of the immune system, akin to macrophages and lymphocytes, use special feelers called "receptors" to recognize invaders or foreign particles. When these scavenger cells sense the build up of too many AGEs, they first remove them, and then get to repairing the damage. The ideal scenario is no scar, no wrinkles, no redness, just smooth, elastic, healthy skin, like that of children's. But when too many AGEs keep coming in, the situation turns to harmful inflammation rather than healthy repair. This is when skin health begins to suffer.

Have you noticed that as one gets older simple wounds heal slowly or leave scars that are bigger or darker and bothersome? Aging comes with the accumulation of wrinkled skin, which is bound to be more prominent whenever excess AGEs are brought in with food or smoking.

AGEs from food can end up in a fat layer that normally lies under the skin. This portion of body fat (called subcutaneous fat), like other fat stores in the body, can accumulate oxidized AGE-fat. In the skin, this type of fatty tissue often looks "lumpy" and tends to expand quite rapidly. These lumps, also known as cellulite, are notoriously difficult to "melt away," even after drastic dieting. The reason that they don't respond to dieting is that the weight-loss diets cannot break down AGE-fat. In fact, few chemicals can break AGEs, even in the laboratory. So, it is no wonder that the encouraging results of most diets are often tainted by fat packets stubbornly attached to our abdomen, buttocks, and thighs.

It is easy now to anticipate the pattern: AGEs work on skin in the same ways as they do in arteries, kidneys, the brain, and so on. One way to surely and safely have an impact on your skin, or improve its youthfulness is to lower AGE intake. The AGE-Less Way is a great way to help skin wounds heal faster and with less scarring. This, together with a sense of well being, is hugely important especially to those who have diabetes or are older.

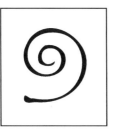

Chapter 6
Coming to Grips with the Issue

It All Begins in the Womb

Certain health conditions can be tracked way back, to the time we spend in the womb. Among the most important examples are diabetes and heart disease. Some of these are now thought to be transmittable, not through genes of either parent, but from the mother to her infant through the blood. Excessive weight gain and obesity prior to pregnancy puts women at risk for diabetes during pregnancy, and these women are also more likely to develop diabetes and high blood pressure. For instance a recent report showed that more than 70% of women with diabetes during their pregnancy had a high pre-pregnancy BMI (greater than 25). The good news is that nearly one half of this type of diabetes (gestational diabetes) can be prevented with weight control. This is an important goal, since diabetes during pregnancy can become permanent and can seriously compromise the mother's health for the rest of her life.

On the other hand, mother-to-child disease transmission has been the subject of extensive research. The mother's blood is a common route of transmission, and is one of the reasons that diseases such as obesity and diabetes now affects people at a younger age. But little is known about the nature of the factors transmitted. For example, everyone knows that women should avoid certain behaviors during pregnancy, such as alcohol and smoking, which can harm the baby.

Until recently, nothing was known about AGEs during pregnancy. This should come as no surprise. It is only very recently that we reported data from a study in sixty mothers and their infants, before and after delivery. As is often the case nowadays, all infants were first breast-fed and then placed on formulas and solid foods. A close relationship in blood AGE levels between mothers and infants was evident at birth, that is, even before tasting their mother's milk. High levels of AGEs in the mother translated into high AGE levels in the infant. Conversely, when the AGE levels were low in the mother, they were also low in the infant. These findings suggested a passive transfer of oxidant AGEs from mother to infant long before the child is born.

As these babies reached 12 months of age, an age at which all had transitioned to infant formulas or solid baby foods, we noted with alarm that by that time levels of blood AGEs had already doubled and even

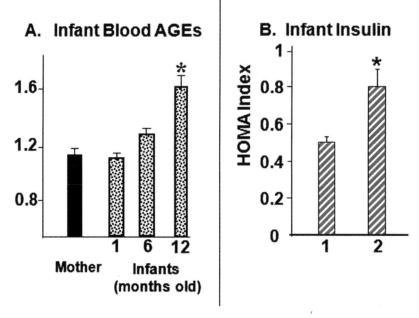

Figure 6: **A.** In infants, blood AGEs can be as high as their mother's (black bar) as soon as they are born and increase rapidly in the first year of life (grey bars). **B.** Insulin levels can be abnormally high in infants of mothers with high blood AGEs (2), compared to infants of mothers with low AGEs (1), spelling danger of diabetes in the child. Message: pregnant women should be aware of their AGE intake and lower it as soon as possible if needed.

exceeded the "adult" levels, in their mother's blood (**Figure 6**). In fact many infants had as high AGEs as adults with diabetes or kidney disease. There were other troubling findings. Many infants with high AGEs had high levels of insulin, a signal that these children could be already struggling with insulin resistance and pre-diabetes. Some had lower levels of a protective, anti-inflammatory protein, called adiponectin. While these data are still new, they are certainly cause for concern. Wouldn't you take it seriously if your child's blood sugar was high? High AGEs are a greater concern.

The explanation for these findings has since become more clear. Human breast milk is rich in nutritious proteins and fat, but it contains only a small amount of AGEs. This makes it a safe nutrient for infants. Commercial formulas are more enriched in nutrients – and so they are considered even more nutritious - but they are also AGE-rich. This is most likely because most commercial formulas are heat-processed in order to pasteurize, condense, evaporate, or pulverize them. Estimates of AGEs in formulas can be more than 100 times above the levels in human breast milk (**Figure 7**). As soon as the infants were weaned off from breast milk and started on commercial formulas, they were suddenly fed far greater amounts of AGEs on a daily basis. Should infants be exposed to this enormous burden of oxidant AGEs, regardless of their many positive attributes? Not to mention that AGE-modified nutrients pouring in during infancy can overwhelm the delicate immune defense system and affect how it will later respond to the modern environment. We have seen how too many AGEs can ignite harmful inflammation, or how they can damage the pancreas that produces insulin, bringing on diabetes. The damage can also surface many years later as cardiovascular or kidney disease (Chapter 3). It is common today to hear complaints about allergies, asthma, autoimmune diseases, i.e. rheumatoid arthritis, as of diabetes or obesity. Only all of these seem to begin at an earlier age than in previous generations. It is almost as if, ever since AGEs began to dominate modern food and life, a list of diseases trails behind that gets longer by the minute.

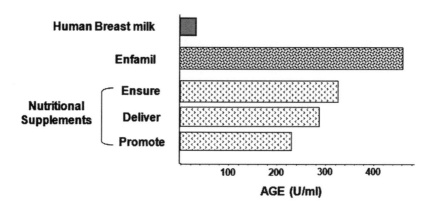

Figure 7: AGE content differs widely among Infant Formulas *(Enfamil)*, nutritional supplements and various feedings, most of which are heat-processed. Note for instance that in *Enfamil* AGEs are over a hundred times higher than in maternal breast milk.

Consider now once more, were you to be told that your child's AGEs were twice the normal level, or that they may become diabetic before reaching the age of twenty: would you be able to ignore it?

Why Now?

Why has it taken so long to recognize AGEs for what they are? Historically, the Western world has come out of a long fight against the specters of hunger, war and economic depression. Throughout long stretches of human history, food came mostly from agricultural crops, scant amounts of meat and modest amounts of fresh dairy foods such as milk, butter, or cheese. So over-consumption of AGEs –largely from animal foods - was quite unlikely. It was infections, lack of sanitation, and famine that robbed humans of the longevity we enjoy today.

The high standard of living in the industrialized western world was built on post-war wealth and the relative abundance of food. New relationships began to take shape between disease and food. Instead of deadly bacteria, a new spectrum of chronic diseases emerged in parallel with the increased production and over-consumption of food. Seeing people who consume several times more than the amounts dictated by the socio-economic norms of the last century is no longer a rarity. Since this is a recent change, the human body could not change so rapidly – it is still designed to handle only a fraction of the loads of AGE toxins brought in by over-eating. This means that it is less able to fight off disease.

The food we eat now is largely processed, exposed to heat, treated with preservatives, colorings, and other flavorings. As a result, appetizing AGEs are now present in high amounts, leading to excessive food intake and thus, excessive AGE consumption.

Although AGEs are as old as the world, AGE toxicity as a result of over-eating, as a problem, is relatively new.

Where From?

Common sense says that the more calories we eat, the more AGEs we consume. But not all foods are equally high in AGEs. For instance, meats and other animal products—even when raw—are a rich source of AGEs, but all else varies a great deal (**Table 6-2**)

Our research has shown that those who eat meat everyday take in four times more AGEs than persons who eat meat two to three times a week. Unfortunately, this conservative estimate applies to much of the American population.

There is a considerable amount of evidence that links disease to meat consumption. Literally hundreds of studies point out the benefits of vegetarian diets. These diets are rich in vegetables, olive oil, and fish, but are low in cheeses, and butter. Studies show that diets containing red meats, or more importantly, high-heat processed (broiled, barbecued, etc.) meats, are especially unhealthy.

Table 6-2: AGE Content in Common Foods Varies with Method of Cooking					
REGULAR DIET				**AGE-LESS DIET**	
Beef:	broiled	5367	→	STEWED	2000
Chicken:	broiled	5245	→	STEWED	1011
Salmon:	broiled	1348	→	RAW	502
Potato:	fried	822	→	STEAMED	17

The levels of AGE in most foods, not only in *red meats*, depend largely on the method of cooking. In the case of fried potatoes, or French fries, part of the difference is due to added oil. AGE kU per 3 oz food

Having said that about red meat, it is not suggested that poultry or fish must be restricted. These important sources of protein are lower in fat. In addition, excess fat can be easily stripped off these types of meat. This accounts for the fact that the total amount of AGEs in cooked fish and chicken is lower than in beef or pork, but it is still quite plentiful, compared to non-meat foods (see Part 3 and Appendix for many more food items). Here again, the method of cooking is hugely important.

Researchers have recently found that in countries where a Mediterranean diet is common, the health benefits attributed to this famous way of eating depend on how the food is prepared. That is, the gains can be lost when this healthy food is cooked by broiling or frying. This means that factors such as *how much* and for *how long* the heat is applied are critical in determining the benefits or risks to health. From our perspective this makes a lot of sense. Formation of new AGEs depends on the method of preparation and the amount of heat used.

While it is important to consume meats with a low-fat content, this is only part of what you need to know: the amount of AGEs that come from animal products that end up on our plate also depends on how the animals were raised, and whether they were fed organic food or com-mercially prepared high-fructose feed based on products with a high content of corn. Animal feeds that are high in fructose are bound to be loaded with AGEs. As you may recall, fructose is at least ten times more efficient in forming AGEs than plain glucose. At the end of the day, how foods are processed before they get to our kitchen, and finally, how we cook them are all important pieces of this new health puzzle that we must still master.

Incidentally, by no means do we suggest doing entirely away with cooking, since to do so would reduce digestibility and increase the risk of spoilage, bacteria, and parasites. What we do encourage however is changing cooking methods. This is far easier than it sounds.

Chapter 7
Learning What to Look For

Values that Matter

Knowing how to control AGEs requires knowing how to measure them. For decades, scientists have been trying to nail down a practical method that allows the measurement of AGEs present in our body, and in our food. Just as we have tools to test blood sugar and cholesterol, we needed reliable tools to assess AGEs. This has been more challenging than anticipated, in part because there a large number of chemical compounds that fall under the general category of AGEs. Some are colorful or fluorescent and are easy to detect, but many others are not, while some are hidden and difficult to access.

The most precise methods are chromatographic or mass spectrophotometric methods, which separate individual compounds by their size, shape, or electric charge. These techniques are expensive and labor intensive. By their nature, they are not yet suitable for application in hospitals, clinics, or commercial food establishments.

Recently, easier methods have become available. Tests for everyday practice are based on the use of antibodies, which are special proteins that recognize common AGEs. The amount of AGEs in these tests has been validated in large numbers of foods and samples of tissues from animals and humans. It took many years before we confirmed that AGEs found in our foods are the same as those in animals and in humans.

Since most AGEs come from food, testing is done in the morning before eating. Using these tests, it was shown that the amount of AGEs in blood accurately reflects the amount in tissues, much like levels of glucose or lipids. Based on many hundreds of blood tests from persons of all ages, races, ethnicities, and both genders, we learned that AGE levels in the fasting state normally range at 6-10 units of AGE per milliliter of blood (U/ml). After a large meal, levels may temporarily double to 15-20 U/ml blood. This is about the level present in a person with diabetes or with high blood cholesterol. Even higher values, up to 25 to 40 U/ml are seen in persons with chronic kidney disease. It is important to remember that such high levels are not too rare today, even among young healthy people, especially if they habitually consume AGE-rich foods. Conversely, it is important to mention here that within two to four months of following the AGE-Less Way, can lower AGEs back to the normal range, along with a stronger constitution against disease.

The bottom line is that we can finally measure AGEs in blood and urine samples. This is the first and most important step in the right direction.

Quick Fixes – None Yet

Yes, there are several drugs that can erase AGEs and their actions. More than thirty years ago, the journal *Science* reported on the first drug found to inhibit AGEs from forming: *aminoguanidine.* This drug became an instant star and was hailed as the new fountain of youth. Subsequent studies led to more effective anti-AGE agents that protected the heart and kidneys in laboratory animals against diabetes and aging. These studies provided concrete evidence at least in one sense: that AGEs are toxic to humans. Unfortunately, most of these drugs got

---

Table 7-1: Potential Anti-AGE Therapies

- **Anti-AGE Agents:**

  - AGE-Inhibitors: Aminoguanidine-HCl, Thiamine-PP, Pyridoxamine (B6), et al.

  - AGE-Breakers: PTB, ALT-711

  - Molecules that sweep up AGEs: sRAGE, Lysozyme, anti-AGE antibodies

- **Anti-Oxidants, Radical Scavengers:**

  - Vitamin E, α-lipoic acid

only as far as animal testing. A few short-term studies went on in humans, but large definitive clinical trials are many years away. Why? Not an easy question to answer. Here is a better one: can we afford to wait? The same question is raised for many other chronic conditions. Whether for heart disease, high blood pressure, stroke or diabetes, many drugs exist but their effects are not sufficiently good. They would probably be far more effective if they were combined with a strategy that deals with the major roadblock, the oxidant overload. The AGE-Less Way may well be the best way to take a big chunk of AGEs right off the top. Why waste this chance?

Why Read This Book?

Day in and day out, we put more than twice as many AGEs in our stomach than we can handle. The problems due to this bad practice start at any time, even at a very young age, and affect every part of the body. Everyone is affected, yet very few are aware of the danger. This is precisely _why_ everyone should read this book. Because it applies to _Everyone_.

The next most important reason is because this is something that can be mastered, controlled and even reversed. The advice in this book can guide you away from a life pattern that was wrong from the start. As easy as it may be to point fingers, it does not pay off. The number of fast food chains is always on the rise. The tobacco industry will not stop producing cigarettes. Nevertheless, people decided to avoid them. You will soon be able to recognize the danger hiding beneath the allure of AGEs.

> _The number of fast food chains is always on the rise. The tobacco industry will not stop producing cigarettes. Nevertheless, people decided to avoid them. The way to go about this is to begin thinking in that same way: avoid them, take the AGE-Less Way._

From the studies sprinkled throughout this book, it should be clear that AGEs accelerate disease and early aging. It is also clear that AGEs trump genetics. This is important for those who may have a genetic predisposition to a disease. The AGE-Less Way can be trusted to slow down or avert a genetic disease. But it is also important for the great majority of those who do not have "bad" genes, to avoid prolonged exposure to food AGEs.

This book explains the paradox of epidemics like diabetes, heart disease, obesity that threaten not only you, but also your family. You surely must be concerned knowing that your family's fate is to live in the midst of them. You probably do not know when to begin worrying, or what to do about it. AGEs are a key factor: they are harmful, universal, man-made, and ushered – rather, forced - into our environment in vast quantities. This is why you should know about AGEs.

You should also know that there is a way out. The AGE-Less Way builds up your core health and keeps you at a safe distance from illness. Even if you develop some inevitable condition, the AGE-Less Way will reduce oxidants in your body and ease their effects. This step alone can lessen the strain of severe common illnesses, such as diabetes, vascular and kidney disease.

If you have children or plan to become pregnant, it is certain that you will need to know about the AGE toxins in your food. If you or someone dear to you is concerned about losing their memory or their mental and intellectual activities, the best plan of action is to follow the AGE-Less Way program.

The AGE-Less Way stitches together a wide array of seemingly unrelated clues and observations, hidden or misunderstood until now. The adage "*we are what we eat*" may be true, but is no longer adequate. It can now be rephrased to "we are *how we prepare* what we eat."

When to Begin?

The build up of AGEs begins with our first meal or rather, in our mother's womb. The body can handle small amounts of AGEs. However, as with all toxins, it cannot handle a constant excess of AGEs throughout our life. The AGE-Less Way is most effective if started at a young age, when eating habits are being established. Besides, AGEs are trans-ferred during pregnancy from the mother to the unborn child. So it is never too early for you and your children to get started on the AGE-Less Way.

By the same token, it is never too late to start the AGE-Less Way. You can immediately see improvement by simply reducing the toxic burden added with your food. Starting today will surely lighten the pressure on your over-extended natural defenses and allow your kidneys to excrete AGEs that have built up in your tissues. This will strengthen your protec-tive reserves, fend off disease and, ultimately, will slow down the rate at which you age.

So, anytime is a good time to begin. The old phrase, *"better late than never"* definitely applies here.

PART 2:

Plan Your AGE-Less Way:
From Principles to Practice

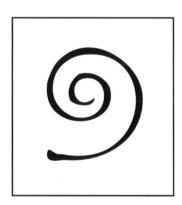

Chapter 8
Mastering the AGE-Less Way

Basic Principles

As we learned, a key to how well we live—or age—could depend on how many AGEs we consume with food every day. By reducing AGEs in your diet, you could skip or postpone trouble and disease associated with aging. This chapter will help you understand how to master the AGE-Less Way. It comes down to knowledge of four basic steps, which can be applied whether eating at home or at a restaurant:

1. Avoid high-AGE foods and food groups.
2. Choose cooking methods that prevent the formation of AGEs.
3. Avoid food combinations that foster the formation of AGEs.
4. Use ingredients that deter the formation of AGEs.

It is important to remember that you do not have to totally eliminate foods that contain AGEs. We just have to reduce the amount we consume by about half. By keeping dietary AGEs to a reasonable level, your body can safely handle and eliminate them without being overwhelmed. This is the whole secret: learning how to choose and prepare AGE-Less foods is simple and can save you money. You will not have to eliminate your favorite foods, suffer through tasteless meals, eat only raw foods, or go hungry. Just as important, the AGE-Less Way can be enjoyed by the entire family.

STEP 1 – Avoid High-AGE Foods

Animal protein poses one of the biggest problems for us. The reasons? Meat, especially red meat, contains preformed AGEs that rise to even higher levels during cooking. Another big concern is fat, especially butter, but also margarine and vegetable oils. AGEs form in fats during refining and processing and increase even more during cooking. On the other hand, vegetables, fruits, whole grains, and milk are naturally low in AGEs. Be aware though, when grains are processed into crispy brown or fatty snack foods and sweetened with sugar or honey, their AGE content can be quite high. Milk too, when processed into cheese, can become very high in AGEs.

Four Easy Steps:
1. *Avoid high-AGE foods.*
2. *Choose cooking methods that prevent the formation of AGEs.*
3. *Avoid food combinations that foster the formation of AGEs.*
4. *Use ingredients that deter the formation of AGEs.*

So how do you balance your diet to keep dietary AGEs within reasonable limits? The first step is to keep meat portions modest. Secondly, adopt a leaner, less processed diet. Just by doing this, you will automatically sidestep many of the foods that are highest in AGEs. Practically speaking, simply limit portions of animal protein to no more than one quarter of the lunch or dinner plate. Then fill the remainder of the plate with fresh, steamed, or lightly sautéed vegetables; whole grains; and fruits. These recommendations have been tested by large numbers of people before you, and are no different from wise advice given to prevent heart disease, cancer, diabetes, and many other health problems. Now you have another important reason for doing so.

Table 8-1 provides a general guide to foods according to AGE content. AGEs are measured in kilounits (kU). On the AGE-Less Way, you should aim for 5,000 to 8,000 kU of AGEs per day. In the following chapters, you will learn much more about putting your AGE-Less Way plan into action whether in your own kitchen or when eating away from home. For an expanded list of foods, see Appendix.

Table 8-1: AGE Categories for Selected Foods*

Very-low: (< 100 kU/serv)	Fresh, plain frozen, canned, and cooked vegetables Fresh, plain frozen, and canned (in water or juice) fruits Low-fat breads, such as bagels, pita bread, sandwich-type breads and rolls Minimally processed cereals such as oatmeal, shredded wheat, and bran flakes Boiled or steamed rice and other whole grains Popcorn without butter Milk, yogurt, soy milk Eggs – poached, scrambled, or steam-basted Canned vegetable and bean soups, chicken and beef bouillon and broth Nonfat mayonnaise and salad dressings, mustard, soy sauce, vinegar Frozen fruit pops, sorbet, gelatin, ice cream, pudding Coffee, tea, wine
Low: (100 – 500 kU/serv)	Toasted breads Pasta Low-fat bran muffin Cooked or canned dried beans, peas, and lentils Canned tuna (water-packed) Avocado, olives Mayonnaise and salad dressing (low-fat or light) Vegetarian burgers, vegetarian sausage, and vegetarian bacon
Medium: (501 – 1,000 kU/serv)	Cereal bars, granola bars Hummus Poached or boiled chicken Poached or steamed fish Canned salmon (water-packed) Low-fat and light natural cheeses such as mozzarella, Swiss, and cheddar Dark chocolate Sunflower and pumpkin seeds (raw) Some vegetable oils and margarines
High: (1,001 – 2,500 kU/serv)	French fries (fast food) Donuts, pies, cakes, pastries Toasted frozen pancakes or waffles Beef stew, meat balls, meat loaf, burger patty Cheese - processed and full-fat varieties Nuts, peanut butter Butter, mayonnaise (full-fat varieties), some vegetable oils
Very High: (2,501 – 4,000 kU/serv)	Fast food single cheeseburger Broiled or sautéed tofu Broiled, grilled, or fried fish
Exceptionally high: (>4,000 kU/serv)	Roasted, grilled, or fried beef, pork, poultry Fast food double cheeseburger, chicken nuggets Hot dog, sausage, bacon Pizza

*AGE content is based on typical manufacturer suggested serving sizes. For instance, the serving size for most breakfast cereals is 2 ounces, meats 3 ounces, cheese 1 ounce, margarine or butter 1 tablespoon, etc. So if you eat more than the suggested serving size, you get more AGEs.

STEP 2 – Choose Cooking Methods that Reduce New AGEs

The AGE-Less Way focuses on preparation. While some foods natu-rally contain AGEs, it is the way they are prepared that ultimately determines their AGE content. The concept is simple: the main cause for the rise of AGEs in food is high, dry heat. The best way to avoid an excess of AGEs is to cook at a lower temperature with lots of moisture. Any kind of cooking that uses a lot of heat and browns the outside of food means that the food will contain toxic levels of AGEs. Thus, cooking food by methods such as searing, browning, grilling, roast-ing, and frying should be minimized. This echoes recommendations from the American Cancer Society, which advises consumers to avoid charring because it produces carcinogenic chemicals known as het-erocyclic amines (HCAs).

What are the best ways to produce a low amount of AGEs during cooking? Moist heat methods, such as poaching, steaming, and stewing. These cooking methods are very much in tune with the needs of the average working household because they are simple and fast. So you can enjoy healthy, low-fuss meals with no need for fancy and cumbersome cooking methods. You will find many delicious ways to use these AGE-Less cooking techniques in the recipe section of this book (Part 3).

Keep in mind that the key is to cut back on the heat and increase moisture, not to completely eliminate a cooking technique that you like. If you love a certain barbecued or roasted dish, save it for special occa-sions when you eat out or grill. Similarly, Thanksgiving only comes once a year, so there is no reason to give up that perfectly browned turkey.

You can also look for lower-AGE ways to satisfy a taste for grilled or roasted foods, such as grilled or roasted vegetables and fruits. While a roasted caramelized pear contains more AGEs than a poached pear, the total amount is still small relative to a piece of roasted meat. You might also have a grilled sandwich or quesadilla made with vegetables, tuna, poached chicken and low-fat cheese fillings. Again, the amount of AGEs in the grilled bread or tortilla is a lot less than that of grilled meat.

Comparing Cooking Methods

The same amount of raw food can give rise to greater or fewer AGEs depending on whether the food is cooked with dry or moist heat, how long it is cooked, and how high the temperature is set. The following chart compares the AGE content of chicken prepared by various cooking methods. Keep in mind that the AGE-Less Way recommends consuming 5,000 to 8,000 kU AGEs per day.

Chicken	AGEs (kU per 3-oz. serving)
Raw	700
Poached or boiled	1,000
Roasted	4,300
Broiled	5,250
Deep fried	6,700
Chicken nuggets (fast food)	8,000

[Reference: Goldberg, T. et al; *Journal of the American Dietetic Association* 2004;104:1287-91.]

Tip: While cooking methods, such as roasting and broiling, rapidly cause AGEs to form, moist heat methods such as poaching or stewing are much more forgiving. For instance, a piece of chicken simmered for 15-20 minutes has a lot less AGEs than chicken broiled for the same amount of time.

Tips for Heating Leftovers and Pre-cooked Foods
Whether cooking or reheating food, the level of heat generated and the amount of time that the food is exposed to heat determines its AGE content. This also goes for reheating leftovers and warming pre-cooked foods. For food safety reasons, it is recommended that leftovers be reheated to 165 degrees F. Soup, sauces, and gravies should

be brought to a boil. Leftover soup or stew can simply be reheated on a stovetop. Since these foods contain a lot of water, AGE formation will be minimal during reheating. Foods such as leftover pot roast can be reheated in a covered pot on the stovetop along with some of the pot roast juices or sauce. Microwave is best for reheating foods (for a short time) with plenty of liquid, just to the desirable temperature.

STEP 3 – Avoid Food Combinations that Foster AGEs

The combination of foods is an important, but more complex aspect of AGE chemistry. In addition to containing its own preformed AGEs, meat presents an additional problem when combined with certain foods in the same meal. This is because proteins and fats in meat can react with sugars in the meat itself or in other foods to create more new AGEs. The reason is simple: cooking foods rich in oxidized fats or proteins sets up chain reactions that form more and more AGEs, resulting in a flood of oxidants that end up in the bloodstream. The following combinations are "*hot*" sources of AGEs and should be avoided:

> meat + foods high in sugar
> meat + high-fat or processed cheeses
> meat + butter, bacon, or sausage

For example, when you eat a hamburger, you are taking in AGEs (which are present in the meat) that go directly into your bloodstream. If you top that burger with bacon and cheese, you may stimulate the production of more AGEs during the process of digestion and absorption, and then in the bloodstream. If you follow that burger with a piece of cake, then you are setting up a situation where the proteins and fats in the meat and cheese get to react with the sugars in the cake to create even more AGEs. As was previously explained, this is because AGEs set up chain reactions with other oxidized components in the diet. It is best then to avoid these *hot* combinations as much as possible or minimize them by choosing better replacements, such as low-fat unprocessed cheese and low-fat or vegetarian bacon or sausage. It is also important to keep portions moderate so they do not provide excess proteins and sugars to form additional AGEs.

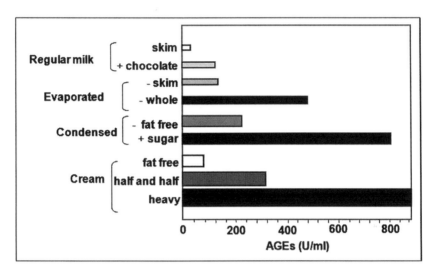

Figure 9: Most foods contain some AGEs before you begin to cook. This initial amount will generally increase, during cooking, depending on the method you use, that is, temperature, time and water present. Microwaving must be kept brief, and is best when used for liquids.

STEP 4— How to Deter AGEs

As discussed earlier in this chapter, new AGE formation increases under certain cooking conditions such as high-dry heat or by combining certain foods or ingredients. This means that cooking with moist heat offers protection by keeping AGE formation low (**Figure 9 and table on page 81**). Another great protective agent that you should know about is acid. AGEs are discouraged from forming in an acidic environment such as lemon juice, red wine, or vinegar (**Figure 10**)— which brings us to the topic of marinades.

Magical Marinades
Marinades that contain acidic ingredients like vinegar, lemon, or tomato juice can suppress AGE formation in meats, poultry, and

seafood during high-temperature cooking such as barbecuing, broil-ing, or grilling. Marinating meats for even a couple of hours prior to cooking can prevent AGE formation by a good fifty percent. Of course it all depends on the thickness of the meat and the amount of acidic liquid around it. Small meat surfaces and large volumes of liquid are the best. Here are some specific guidelines for marinating food to reduce AGEs.

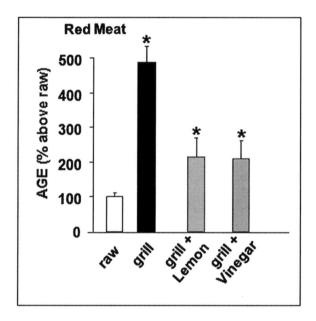

Figure 10: To prevent some of the AGEs that form on meats during cooking, like grilling (black bar) you can marinate them in an acidic liquid like lemon juice or vinegar (gray), or tomato juice for anywhere between 1 hr and 12 hours.

Tips for AGE-Less Marinades
- For one pound of meat, use the juice from two lemons (about 4 to 6 tablespoons) or an equivalent amount of vinegar or lime juice plus enough water to cover the food (about 1 cup). Bottled lemon juice is okay. For extra flavor, add seasonings like garlic, ginger, pepper, capers, and fresh or dried herbs.
- Use a non-reactive container or zip-top plastic food bag to hold the meat and marinade.

- Avoid commercial marinades or marinade recipes that are high in sugar and/or oil. Salad dressings such as light balsamic vinaigrette or light Italian are convenient options for marinades.
- Marinate the food for at least 1 hour or up to 12 hours.

Table 8-2 lists some common acidic foods that you might want to use in marinades or cooking. The term "pH" is a measure of how basic or acidic a substance is based on a scale of 0 to 14. A pH of 7 is considered neutral. Values greater than 7 are more basic (alkaline), while values less than 7 are more acidic. AGEs form readily at a pH above 7, but are retarded at a pH below 7.

Table 8-2: pH of some common foods*

Food	pH
Buttermilk	4.4- 4.8
Lemon juice	2.0 – 2.6
Lime juice	2.0 – 2.8
Mustard	3.5 – 6.0
Wine	3.3 – 3.7
Soy sauce	4.4 – 5.4
Tomatoes, canned	3.5 – 4.7
Vegetable juice	3.9 – 4.3
Vinegar	2.4 – 3.4

*Source: http://www.cfsan.fda.gov/~comm/lacf-phs.html

Tip: While acidic marinades help prevent AGEs, they also help tenderize meats and poultry. In addition, sour ingredients like lemon juice and vinegar reduce the need for adding salt. So now you have several reasons to marinade meats and poultry whenever possible.

Giving Your Recipes an AGE-Less Make Over

Many of your favorite recipes can be easily modified to reduce AGEs. Learning about the foods and techniques presented in the first part of this chapter is the first step toward preparing AGE-Less meals. The following table (Table 8-3) offers additional tips for transforming your favorite recipes into new AGE-Less versions.

Table 8-3: How to Change AGEs

Type of Recipe	To lower AGEs ...
Burgers	Use lean ground meat. Add some finely chopped mushrooms and other vegetables to the burger mixture. This will increase moisture, boost nutritional value, and make meat portions go further. Shape the center of burgers slightly thinner than the edges. This will promote faster, more even cooking. Avoid pressing down on the burgers during cooking, as this will remove moisture. Cook on nonstick surfaces such as a nonstick skillet or a tabletop grill such as a George Foreman grill with a nonstick coating. (Direct contact with a steel cooking or grilling surface enhances AGE formation.)
Meatballs	Use lean ground meat. Use fresh untoasted bread crumbs instead of dried toasted crumbs. Omit the browning step and simmer the meatballs in the sauce until cooked through.
Meatloaf	Use lean ground meat. Use fresh untoasted bread crumbs or oatmeal instead of dried toasted crumbs. Add lots of finely chopped vegetables to meatloaf mixtures to boost nutritional value, add moisture, and make meat portions go further.
Soups & stews	Include acidic ingredients like tomatoes or wine in the cooking liquid. Note that if too much of an acidic ingredient is used, grains and vegetables may toughen and not cook properly. Minimize or omit the browning step.
Grilled meats	Marinate the meat in acidic liquid for 1 to 12 hours before grilling. Wrap meats in a foil pouch for the first part of cooking, or pre-cook the meat until almost done by poaching or steaming. Finish cooking the last few minutes on a nonstick grill surface. Steaks and roasts cooked rare or medium-rare will have lower amounts of AGEs than well-done meats. However, always be sure to follow food safety precautions for cooking meat. (See the latter part of the chapter for safe cooking temperature recommendations.)

Salads	For main dish salads, add poached chicken, steamed seafood, or legumes instead of grilled or roasted chicken and meat. Use unprocessed reduced-fat cheeses. Use low-fat or light mayonnaise and salad dressings. Substitute canned chickpeas or kidney beans for croutons. Or toss in some leftover cooked penne or rotini pasta. Instead of having crackers as an accompaniment to a salad, enjoy wedges of whole grain pita bread.
Omelets, frittatas	Use more whites and fewer yolks, or choose a fat-free egg substitute. Use unprocessed reduced-fat cheese. When making cheese-topped frittatas, sprinkle the cheese on last and cook just long enough to melt. Do not brown the cheese.
Casseroles	If the recipe includes browned ground beef or turkey, cook it in a covered skillet to retain moisture and minimize browning. If the recipe calls for cooked chicken, use poached chicken instead of grilled or roasted. Use unprocessed, reduced-fat cheese and add any cheese toppings only during the last minute of cooking—just long enough to melt. Do not brown.
Pizza	Feature vegetable toppings instead of high-fat meats like sausage and ground beef. Use low-fat or part-skim mozzarella cheese and add it only during the last minute or two of cooking—just long enough to melt. Do not brown.
Sandwiches	Use lower-AGE fillings like poached chicken, canned tuna or salmon, or egg instead of roasted or grilled meats. Limit the amount of meat in sandwiches to a couple of ounces. Add bulk with lots of lettuce, tomato, onion, and other vegetables. Use low-fat or light spreads and dressings. Use reduced-fat unprocessed cheeses. When making grilled sandwiches, lightly coat the outside of the bread with cooking spray instead of spreading with butter or margarine.

Cook it Safely

To minimize AGEs, it is important to not overcook food. You also want to be careful that certain foods reach proper temperatures for food safety reasons. The USDA recommends using a food thermometer for checking "doneness" of meats, seafood, and poultry. These foods should be cooked to these safe minimum internal temperatures.

Beef, lamb, or pork steaks, roasts, and chops - 145 °F with a 3-minute rest time (i.e. let the meat sit for 3 minutes after removing from heat source).
Fish - 145 °F
Ground beef, lamb, or pork - 160 °F
Egg Dishes - 160 °F
Poultry (whole, pieces, or ground) - 165 °F

References:
http://www.fsis.usda.gov/is_it_done_yet/
http://www.foodsafety.gov

Starting On the AGE-Less Way – The Sooner, The Better

You can easily lower AGEs to manageable levels by choosing AGE-Less ingredients and cooking methods, and by avoiding the "hot" food combinations discussed earlier in this chapter. Keep in mind that the AGE-Less Way should be the eating choice for all members of the family.

Scientific evidence shows that the AGE-Less Way can and should be started at a young age, when eating habits are being established. In fact, as discussed in Chapter 6, the AGE-Less Way should start with the mother's diet during pregnancy. This means that the mother can make sure that the baby's AGE exposure is as low as possible, and this will make for a healthier newborn. The following chapters provide additional tips for implementing the AGE-Less Way—anywhere and anytime.

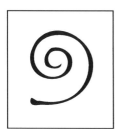

Chapter 9
AGE-Less Eating Away
From Home

Choosing a Restaurant

Eating out is one of the pleasures of life. It can be even more so while on the AGE-Less Way because not only do you enjoy your meals more, but you also develop a sense of healthier well-being. Restaurants and stores that sell fast foods, take-out, and convenience foods that are high in AGEs have become so popular that many people have literally replaced home cooking. The only way to apply the AGE-Less Way when eating out is to choose very carefully. However, an increasing number of restaurants today present delicious choices that are low in AGEs. This chapter will help you make the most of the menu in a wide variety of settings.

General Tips

Unlike home-prepared meals, it's not always possible (if not almost impossible today) to know exactly what you are getting when you eat out, especially about AGEs. However, until the amount of AGEs appears on food labels, a few general tips can go a long way toward managing your AGE intake when eating away from home.

-Be Wise about Size
We frequently ingest too many AGEs simply because we eat too much food, and super-sized restaurant food is a big part of the problem.

Eating oversized portions can overload the body with preformed AGEs, along with sugar, fat, and calories. As we discussed, AGEs form from mixing sugar, fat, and proteins together during cooking and greater amounts of these ingredients will create even more AGEs in the digestive system that can then enter the bloodstream. Use these tips to deal right away with the restaurant-size portions. These solutions are both smart and simple, like getting two for the price of one:

- Ask if you can order a smaller (i.e. reasonable) portion. Some restaurants offer half-portions or "senior" portions for a reduced price.
- Split the main course with someone or take half of it home for another meal.
- Dine out more often for lunch than for dinner. Portions (and prices) tend to be substantially smaller at lunch as they are at dinner. This allows you to cut down on AGEs and save money too.
- Create a meal out of appetizers and side dishes, such as a shrimp cocktail with salad and a cup of vegetable soup.
- Choose bigger portions of vegetables and salads, moderate portions of starchy foods (like whole grains, beans, potatoes) and fruits, and smaller portions of meat and cheese.
- As a general guideline, plant foods should cover about three quarters of the lunch or dinner plate.
- Ask for olive oil, rather than butter; a dash of oregano adds a lot of flavor to the oil.

-Choose poached, steamed, stewed, or boiled main courses

We generally choose one meat course when we eat out. It could be red meat, chicken, or fish. As you know by now, meats—especially grilled, broiled, seared, roasted, and fried meat—are the primary contributors to an overload of AGEs. A huge advantage of the AGE-Less Way is that you do not have to go hungry. Nonetheless, meat portions should be kept modest. A major key to success is choosing a preparation method that uses water or moist heat, such as poaching, stewing, steaming, and boiling. Whether dining out or cooking at home, aim to limit red meat to no more than twice a week. Choose more dishes like soups and stews that feature smaller amounts of simmered meat, chicken, or seafood with lots of vegetables. In this way, you will be within the range of AGEs that your body can safely eliminate and ahead of the game with your personal AGE-Less Way.

-Limit desserts and fatty cheeses after a meat meal

When we eat a meal full of meat followed by a sugary dessert or cheese, we create a kind of extended "cooking" in the body. This is because the fat mixes with the extra sugars as they move along our digestive system and are then absorbed in the bloodstream to form even more AGEs. If you have a sugar rich dessert, share it with others and enjoy just a few bites. Even better, opt for an AGE-Less treat such as a small dish of fruit (fresh, poached, roasted, or grilled), sorbet, sherbet, granita, ice cream, frozen yogurt, or pudding.

-Focus on lower-fat foods

Butter, cream, oils, and other processed fats are very high in AGEs. Choose foods made with lower-fat sauces, spreads, and dressings to minimize AGE intake. Another smart move is to request dressings and sauces on the side so you can control how much is added.

-Balance a high-AGE restaurant meal with lower AGE choices throughout the day

If you have grilled or roasted meat at lunch, keep your daily AGE intake in check by choosing lower-AGE foods at other meals. For example, enjoy oatmeal, fruit, and milk for breakfast and have bean soup and salad for dinner.

-Be mindful of mindless eating and drinking

Here is a great catch: creamy-sweet super-sized coffee drinks, sugary sodas, pastries, and other grab-and-go fare can add greatly to your AGE load by delivering high amounts of refined sugars, processed fats, and preformed AGEs. Strangely, many think that snack foods must be something processed to be considered "good." These include "meal replacement" or protein bars, or chips, crackers and cookies. These are highly processed and do not really resemble the natural foods from which they are derived. We must stick to real food and think of snacks as mini-meals that can provide nourishment, when needed, between regular meals. But what is more important here is to remember that processed snack foods are often heat-treated items that are disproportionately rich in AGEs, compared to the amount of AGEs in regular food. So snack smartly with choices like antioxidant-rich fruit, yogurt, or a low-fat latte with a dash of cocoa. For a more substantial snack, have a cup of soup, a small bowl of cereal, or leftovers from a low-AGE meal. Again, think "real food." Chapter 18 offers additional ideas and tips for smart snack choices. Eliminating eating between meals is an excellent solution. One option to control snacking is to chew sugarless gum or keep a sugarless mint in your mouth.

AGE-Less Menu Options

Just about every type of restaurant has some delicious lower-AGE options. In some cases, you may request slight modifications to menu items to lower their AGE content. Helpful hint: try new foods! Many ethnic menus contain low-AGE dishes and can expand your choices to a whole new world of possibilities. Here are some ideas to get you started.

Chinese

Have you ever noticed how few Chinese persons are overweight? There are many reasons for this, but their ways of preparing food is certainly one of them. Chinese dishes, with their ample portions of vegetables and modest portions of meat, are a good example of right-sized portions for AGE-Less meals. Many dishes featured on authentic Chinese menus are also steamed, which is perfect for AGE-Less eating. Another important and useful tip is the Chinese way of quickly passing very thinly sliced meat over the hot pan. This prevents the formation of excessive AGEs, but still makes sure that the meat is thoroughly cooked. Unfortunately, American-style Chinese food is usually higher in fat, heavily sauced, and disproportionately deep-fried. Again, this is exactly how we have become accustomed to eat in this country. So steer clear of the deep-fried egg rolls, fried rice, and fried wontons or foods seasoned with toasted sesame oil (which is very high in AGEs) and choose instead:

- Broth-based soups such as egg drop, hot & sour, and wonton
- Steamed dumplings
- Steamed fish, tofu, and vegetable dishes
- Hot pot meals made with seafood, tofu, or chicken and vegetables (foods cooked at the table fondue-style in a pot of simmering broth)
- Egg foo yung made with seafood, tofu, or vegetables
- Steamed or boiled brown rice
- Steamed or boiled noodles
- Hot mustard, soy sauce, ginger

Tip: Some Chinese restaurants will be happy to steam (rather than stir-fry), many of their dishes. In this case, you could opt for many combinations of seafood or chicken and vegetables. However, stir-fry is still better than American-style deep-fried foods. If you do get a stir-fried dish, choose seafood, tofu, or chicken, which will have about half as many AGEs as stir-fried beef.

Japanese
As with most Asian cuisine, Japanese dishes feature moderate amounts of meat and plenty of vegetables, which fit well with the AGE-Less Way. Examples of lower-AGE dishes include:

- Miso and other broth-based soups with vegetables, seafood, chicken, or noodles
- Sashimi (raw slivered fish)
- Edamame (boiled green soybeans)
- Salads made with seaweed, cucumber, vegetables, or steamed seafood

- Sushi made with seafood (non-fried) or vegetables
- Steamed or boiled vegetable or seafood dumplings
- Boiled soba (buckwheat) noodles or udon (wheat) noodles simmered in broth with vegetables, tofu, or seafood
- Steamed rice (ask if brown rice is available)

French

There is a misguided belief that French people, especially women, remain slim even though they eat a great deal of fatty foods. While French cuisine is perhaps best known for creamy sauces and buttery croissants, it also has a lighter, less caloric side that fits perfectly into your AGE-Less Way. Many classic French dishes use AGE-Less cooking methods such as poaching, braising, and steaming in wine or tomato sauce. Roasted or grilled vegetables may also be featured and are much lower in AGEs than roasted or grilled meats. Remember that great salads are extremely popular as is fresh raw seafood. Here are some items to look for:

- Mussels simmered in tomato, wine, or mustard sauce
- Crab or shrimp cocktail
- Smoked salmon
- Consommé and broth-based soups
- Bean and lentil soups and stews
- Grilled or roasted vegetables
- Steamed or poached seafood and poultry (order sauces on the side)
- Seafood cooked en Papillote (steamed in parchment paper packets)
- Seafood or chicken Provencal (cooked in tomato or tomato-wine sauce)
- Seafood or vegetable stews such as bouillabaisse and ratatouille
- Salads with light vinaigrette dressing or ask for oil and vinegar

Tip: Ask that a minimum of fat be added during food preparation. For instance, adding a couple of teaspoons of butter to a packet of fish cooked en Papillote, could easily triple the AGE content of the dish. Whenever possible, choose olive oil over butter.

Italian

Mediterranean foods are proven over many years and in hundreds of studies to be the healthiest food within the European family of diets. Southern Italian cuisine is one of them. Pasta in moderation is a great low-AGE staple. Pair it with red sauce, a glass of red wine, and plenty of colorful veggies to punch up meals with health promoting phytonutrients. Keep in mind that gobs of melted cheese and piles of Parmesan will quickly put you over your AGE limit, so go easy on the cheese. Here are some lower-AGE items that you might find on the menu.

- Vegetable and bean soups like pasta fagioli and minestrone
- Steamed clams or mussels in tomato or wine sauce
- Pasta with tomato sauce such as arrabbiata, marinara, and puttanesca
- Pasta with red clam sauce
- Seafood Fra Diavolo (in a spicy red sauce)
- Seafood stews such as cioppino
- Garden salad with vinaigrette dressing
- Grilled or roasted vegetables
- Cappuccino made with low-fat milk

Greek

Among Mediterranean foods, Greek and Portuguese cuisines have been identified as the best, since these countries were among those with the lowest rates of major diseases, like heart disease and diabetes. Unfortunately, this may no longer be true since the high-fat, high-AGE "American" type of diet has been spreading everywhere. Still, the original principles are there for us to make good use of: olive oil rather than butter, vegetable-based main courses rather than meats, fresh fish rather than fatty red meats. Many Greek dishes feature flavorful herbs, yogurt, lemon, beans, seafood, and vegetables. Enjoy these often on your AGE-Less Way. Save the buttery filo-crusted pies and roasted meats for an occasional indulgence. Keep in mind that feta sold in the United States is high in AGEs, probably due to extra pasteurization, so have just a sprinkling. Fortunately, a little bit of this flavorful cheese can go a long way. Some lower-AGE items that you may find on menus include:

- Dips and spreads made with vegetables, beans, and yogurt such as tzatzikí (yogurt, cucumber, garlic and herbs), and melintzano-salata (eggplant spread with garlic, olive oil, and lemon)
- Soups such as avgolemono (egg, lemon and rice in chicken broth), fasoláda (white bean and vegetable), lentil, and seafood
- Baked fish dishes such as Plaki (fish baked with tomatoes, onions, and garlic) and fish baked in grape leaves
- Dolmades—seasoned ground meat and rice wrapped in grape-vine leaves
- Lamb marinated with Greek herbs, garlic, and lemon
- White beans baked with tomatoes and herbs
- Pita sandwiches with grilled or roasted eggplant, portabella, zucchini, and other vegetables
- Greek salad topped with steamed seafood and a light sprinkling of feta
- Pita bread

Middle Eastern

Encompassing many different countries and a wide range of cuisines, Middle Eastern fare has many tasty AGE-Less selections to offer. Bulgur wheat, chickpeas, eggplant, yogurt, olive oil, parsley, and aromatic herbs and spices are among the many healthful foods featured. Some AGE-Less items that you may find on menus include:

- Vegetable and bean dips and spreads such as hummus (blended chickpeas with tahini, lemon, olive oil, and seasonings) and baba ghanouj (roasted eggplant with lemon, olive oil, tahini, garlic, and herbs)
- Soups and stews made with lentils, chickpeas, fava beans, vegetables, seafood, chicken, and lamb

- Wraps and pitas with hummus, baba ghanouj, or falafel (Falafel patties are traditionally deep-fried, but some restaurants may bake them upon request.)
- Tabbouleh salad (bulgur wheat with tomatoes, cucumber, lemon, olive oil, and parsley)
- Stuffed cabbage rolls with rice and ground chicken or lamb
- Couscous with stewed vegetables, beans, seafood, chicken, or lamb

Indian

Like Mediterranean and Middle Eastern food, Indian cuisine is rich in vegetables, lamb, and, most importantly, herbs and spices. This is a valuable point, since much of the flavor that we crave for and is due to AGEs could be satisfied by a smart use of herbs and spices. Authentic Indian cuisine showcases many delicious vegetarian options that are compatible with AGE-Less Way eating. Generous use of antioxidant-rich spices provides health benefits as well as unique flavors and aromas. Roasted and grilled poultry and meats are also included in many dishes. While they may be low in fat, portions should be kept modest to limit AGE intake. Best bets include:

- Dal (bean, pea, or lentil) stews, soups, or patties
- Broth- or bean-based soups with vegetables, seafood, or chicken
- Chapati and roti (whole wheat flatbreads)
- Raita (cold yogurt-based side dish with cucumbers or other vegetables)
- Chutney (spicy accompaniment to meals), pickles, onion salad
- Vegetable and seafood dishes such as curry or vindaloo (a spicy dish that may include tomato, vinegar, and wine)
- Biriyani (rice dishes) made with vegetables or seafood (Ask if brown rice is available.)

Tip: When ordering, ask that a minimum of fat be used in preparation, as some chefs can have a heavy hand with ingredients like ghee (clarified butter), coconut milk, and oil.

Mexican

From deep-fried tortilla chips to piles of melted cheese, Mexican dining can be a challenge on the AGE-Less Way. Fortunately, many Mexican restaurants are now offering a good selection of vegetarian and lighter options. Most also have an excellent a la carte menu, which allows you to create a meal to suit your needs. Possibilities include:

- Marinated seafood salad such as ceviche and shrimp cocktail
- Broth-based or vegetable soups such as chicken tortilla soup and chilled gazpacho
- Posole (hominy stew) with vegetables or chicken
- Black bean soup, pinto beans
- Bean burrito or enchilada with red or green sauce
- Spinach, vegetable, or seafood enchilada with red or green sauce
- Shrimp or fish tacos in soft corn tortillas
- Grilled vegetable fajitas
- Grilled or roasted vegetables
- Garden salads with light dressing
- Soft (non-fried) corn or wheat tortillas (ask if whole wheat are available)

Tip: Melted cheese is extremely high in AGEs, so go easy on the cheese toppings. Top dishes like burritos and enchiladas with crisp shredded lettuce, diced tomatoes or salsa, and a spoonful of guacamole. Opt for red sauce or verde (green) sauce instead of cheese or sour cream sauces.

Sensational Salads

Crisp, fresh salads are loaded with antioxidants and other important nutrients, making them key to any anti-AGE and anti-aging plan. But do take care when ordering or you might end up with a lot more calories, fat, and AGEs than you bargained for. Whether you are ordering a main dish salad from the menu or creating your own salad at a salad bar, there are plenty of ways to create a salad that is both healthful and delicious.

- *From the menu*—For the lowest-AGEs, choose main dish salads topped with steamed, poached, or lightly grilled shrimp, scallops, or fish (i.e. cooked until done, but not overdone). If what exactly you are looking for is not on the menu, peruse the menu for side dishes, entrees, and ingredients that could perhaps be added to your particular salad. Examples include grilled or roasted vegetables, edamame, assorted beans (lima, cannellini, black, etc.), hard-boiled eggs, or tuna packed in spring water.
- *At the salad bar*—Always start with a pile of fresh spinach or romaine lettuce and plenty of fresh colorful veggies. Add chickpeas, kidney beans, or steamed seafood for protein. Opt for light dressing or a drizzle of vinaigrette dressing. Avoid mayonnaise-based salads such as tuna salad or cole slaw; they are most likely prepared with large amounts of full-fat dressing. Go easy on oily marinated vegetables, draining off as much of the marinade as possible before putting them on the plate. Finish off with some fresh fruit for dessert.

The Reward

As you can see, living the AGE-Less lifestyle does not require that you stay at home and cook all of your own meals. On the contrary, many delicious foods are available for your dining pleasure. We emphasize that the guidelines and tips offered in this chapter and throughout the book are compatible with established guidelines for preventing and treating diabetes, heart disease, cancer, obesity, and many other health problems. They do, however, add a new and critical dimension: reducing exposure to AGEs. As a result, you can maximize the effectiveness of your own health care regimen.

Chapter 10
Stocking the AGE-Less Pantry

Now that you understand the basics of mastering the AGE-Less Way, it's time to put principles into practice. This chapter highlights specific foods featured in the AGE-Less Way, offers smart substitutions for high-AGE foods and ingredients, and provides additional tips for preparing foods.

As you shop for food, keep in mind that the AGE content of the Western diet has increased vastly in the past fifty years due to the excessive processing that many foods now undergo. Processed foods are often exposed to heating and/or dehydration, and both treatments increase the reactions between sugars, proteins and fats in foods to create AGEs. A common theme that you will note throughout this book is that the healthiest eating plan consists of eating freshly prepared food and using the lowest amount of heat you can in its preparation. In addition, concentrate on eating the least possible amount of processed foods.

You will find that AGE-less eating can be tasty, easy to prepare, and economical. By keeping your pantry, refrigerator, and freezer stocked with the right foods, you will always have the makings of a healthful and delicious meal or snack on hand.

Meats and Meat Substitutes

It bears repeating that animal protein, especially red meat, poses a huge AGE problem. Meats naturally contain AGEs and the amount of AGEs is further increased through cooking. So meat gives you a double dose of AGEs—the one already in the meat, and that which is added by cooking. The good news is that you will find ways to marinate meat prior to cooking and cooking methods that will discourage new AGEs. In the end, you will be able to enjoy meat and have a healthy diet. For instance, just three ounces of animal protein prepared by a high-AGE cooking method can put you over the suggested daily limit of 5,000 to 8,000 kU AGE! But the same amount of meat, when prepared by our plan, keeps AGEs to just a fraction of this (Chapter 8). This means that animal origin, portions, *and* cooking methods are all critical to the amount of AGEs formed. Here are the best bets for the AGE-Less Way:

- Meat and poultry: Choose lower-fat cuts, such as skinless chicken breast, lean ground meat, and stew meat that cook quickly and can be cooked with moist heat. When grilling or broiling, it is critical to marinate meats beforehand (see Chapter 8 for more details).
- Fish and shellfish are lower in AGEs than meat and poultry, so try substituting seafood for meat several times a week. AGE-Less Way cooking methods such as poaching, steaming, and cooking en Papillote (steamed in its own juices in foil or parchment packets) are ideal for seafood.
- Canned tuna and salmon are good AGE-Less Way convenience foods to stock up on.
- Frozen steamed or boiled shrimp: Keep some on hand for a simple addition to pasta dishes and salads.
- Dried beans, peas, and lentils (canned or dried) are an exceptionally healthy AGE-Less Way source of protein. Substitute them for meat often, at least several times a week. Make a hearty bean soup, add them to salads and casseroles, or whip up a zesty bean dip or spread.
- Vegetarian burgers are a great AGE-Less protein food to substitute for meat.
- Eggs, especially the whites, are an AGE-Less source of high-quality protein. Enjoy them poached, steam-basted, scrambled, or in frittatas and omelets. If you are watching your cholesterol,

cholesterol-free egg substitutes such as Egg Beaters are also a good AGE-Less option for making omelets and other recipes.
- Canned chicken or beef broth
- Canned or home-made soups with chicken, beef, beans and lentils

 Should You Fret About Fish?

Fish is a rich source of healthy omega-3 fat and it tends to be much lower in AGEs than meat. For these reasons, we recommend replacing meat with fish and seafood several times a week. However, this advice must be balanced against other concerns, such as mercury or other contaminants in seafood, or the environmental impact of over-fishing. Avoiding mercury is especially important for children and women of childbearing age. So how do you get the benefits, but minimize the risk? Use these tips for choosing seafood:

- *Keep portions to three to four ounces cooked (about the size of a deck of cards or half of a chicken breast). This is plenty of protein for one meal.*
- *Avoid swordfish, king mackerel, shark, and tilefish, which are highest in mercury.*
- *Choose lower-mercury species such as salmon, cod, haddock, pollack, tilapia, shellfish, and canned light tuna.*
- *Children and women of childbearing age should limit fish portions to 12 ounces per week and choose only the lower-mercury species.*
- *Watch for updates to seafood safety guidelines and fda.gov or ewg.org.*

AGE-Less Way Tips for High Protein Foods

- All meats, even the most lean, contain a significant amount of AGEs and AGE precursors. Thus, while leaner is better, it is still important to limit portions of animal protein to no more than one quarter of the lunch or dinner plate. Fill the remainder of the plate with vegetables, whole grains, and fruits.

- Cut down on meat portions by serving meat in a pasta or rice dish, salad, soup, or stew.
- Instead of sausage, add flavor to foods with sausage spices. A bit of fennel seed and dried Italian seasoning will lend Italian sausage flavor to a pasta dish or casserole. Sage and a pinch of red pepper adds pork sausage flavor.

Dairy Foods and Substitutes

Many dairy foods can be enjoyed in the AGE-Less Way, although butter and cream, which are very high in AGEs, should be avoided. A drizzle of extra virgin olive oil can be a delicious alternative to butter. Care must also be taken when choosing and cooking with cheeses, since they are generally very AGE-rich. This gets a lot worse when the fat (butter) in cheese is heated again on our stove. This means that all full-fat and processed cheeses should be avoided. Some "light" cheeses are significantly lower in AGEs. Just be sure not to subject them to long cooking times. Choose the following dairy foods and non-dairy alternatives:

- Milk: Nonfat, low-fat, and even whole milk are low in AGEs. To limit saturated fat, choose nonfat and low-fat most often. However, since all kinds of milk are naturally low in fat, you may opt to splurge a bit and use whole milk in coffee, tea, and recipes to add flavor and body. Remember that cream is very high in AGEs.
- Soymilk
- Low-fat yogurt, plain or flavored (preferably with little or no added sugar).
- Greek-style yogurt has been strained to remove part of the whey (liquid), which creates a creamy thick texture similar to sour cream. Greek yogurt is delicious all by itself or served with fruit. It also makes a healthy alternative to sour cream. Choose nonfat or low-fat brands to trim calories and saturated fat.

- Yogurt cheese: Like Greek yogurt, this cheese has been strained to re-move part of the whey. Yogurt cheese contains less whey than Greek yogurt so it has a thicker consistency, similar to soft cream cheese. Yogurt cheese can easily be made at home (see recipe on page 264).
- Light unprocessed cheeses such as part-skim mozzarella and low-fat cheddar and Swiss. Most full-fat cheeses have 8 to 10 grams of fat per ounce, so look for light cheeses with no more than half this amount. If the cheese is to be melted, add it only during the last minute of cooking, just long enough to melt. Do not brown.
- Pudding, preferably low-sugar or sugar-free
- Low-fat ice cream

AGE-Less Tips For Dairy Foods

- Aged and hard cheeses such as feta and Parmesan are very high in AGEs. Fortunately, a little bit can go a long way, so use just a light sprinkling to add flavor.
- For a low-AGE alternative to cheese, try crumbling a bit of firm raw tofu over salads.
- Spread bagels with a thin layer of nonfat or light cream cheese in-stead of the full-fat version, which is very high in AGEs. Even bet-ter, top bagels with a couple of tablespoons of low-fat Greek-style yogurt or your own homemade yogurt cheese (see page 264).
- Avoid cheeses with labels like "processed cheese," "prepared cheese product," or "cheese food." These cheeses undergo ad-ditional heating, melting, and processing steps, which may raise the AGE content.

Vegetables

Eating plenty of produce is compatible with the AGE-Less Way, since plant foods are naturally low in AGEs. As a bonus, plant foods provide a plethora of age-defying nutrients and antioxidants that help thwart inflammation, oxidation, and AGE formation in the body. Enjoy gen-erous amounts of vegetables at meals and snacks. Choose a rainbow of colors every day to ensure a good assortment of AGE-fighting nutrients (many of which give veggies their vibrant colors). While fresh is best, frozen (without sauce) and canned vegetables are also good.

AGE-Less Tips for Vegetables

- Keep veggies AGE-Less by going easy on added fats. Add just a tablespoon or two of flavorful olive oil to a pan of vegetables instead of drowning them in oil, butter, or cheese sauce as many recipes recommend. Keep in mind that a bit of healthy fat, such as olive oil, is good because it adds flavor and increases the absorption of certain anti-aging antioxidants and phytonutrients in vegetables (such as vitamin E, lycopene, and beta-carotene).
- Eat your veggies unpeeled whenever possible. A high proportion of nutrients and healthy fiber is concentrated in the skin. Just be sure to wash all produce well before cooking and eating.
- Enjoy roasted, broiled, or grilled vegetables. Vegetables prepared this way have more AGEs than steamed vegetables, but the amount is still small compared to the AGEs in roasted or grilled meat.
- For meaty taste and texture, grill or roast portabella mushrooms to enjoy in sandwiches and salads.

 Foods That Fight AGEs

AGEs wreak havoc by triggering inflammation and oxidation. The AGE-Less Way greatly reduces this damage by featuring lower-AGE foods, thus stopping the damage before it starts. You can boost the benefits of your AGE-Less Way plan by choosing more foods with anti-inflammatory and antioxidant powers. What are these foods? Plant foods such as vegetables, fruits, whole grains, legumes, herbs, and spices are chock full of AGE-fighting antioxidants and phytonutrients.

A diet rich in plant foods has been proven time and again to fight off heart disease, cancer, diabetes, and many other health problems. The ability of plant foods to dull the harmful effects of AGEs may be partly responsible for their health benefits, not to mention that plant foods are naturally low in AGEs. So now you have another compelling reason to eat them. Remember the general rule for the AGE-Less Way meal: up to one quarter of the plate can be animal protein and the rest should be vegetables, whole grains, and other plant foods.

Like vegetables, fruits are naturally low in AGEs. Fresh, frozen (without sugar), and canned fruits in juice are featured in the AGE-Less Way program. Dried fruits such as raisins contain more AGEs than fresh fruits, but are still very low on the AGE scale compared to meat. As with vegetables, be sure to choose a variety of colorful fruits to ensure that you are getting a wide array of AGE-fighting antioxidants and phytonutrients.

AGE-Less Tips for Fruits

- Enjoy roasted, grilled, or broiled fruit. A caramelized, baked apple has more AGEs than raw or poached fruit, but is still much lower in AGEs than meat cooked with these methods. So you can choose your "cheats" from the fruit and vegetable categories and still indulge in a tasty treat.
- Purchase fresh, locally grown, in-season produce when possible. It's tastier, likely to be more nutritious, and better for the environment too.
- Eat fruits unpeeled whenever possible. A high proportion of nutrients and healthy fiber is concentrated in the skin. Just be sure to wash all produce well before cooking and eating.
- Get in the habit of having a small dish of fruit for dessert or snack instead of cakes, pies, cookies, and other concentrated sweets. This helps keep blood sugar levels down, causing fewer AGEs to form in the bloodstream.

Breads, Cereals, and Grains

A wide variety of breads, cereals, and grains may be enjoyed on the AGE-Less Way program. Always choose whole grains when possible to boost your intake of AGE-fighting nutrients and antioxidants, which are concentrated in the grain's bran and germ—the parts that are discarded during refining. As a bonus, fiber-rich whole grains help prevent blood sugar levels from surging. Stay away from high-fat and overly processed baked goods and choose from the following:

- Whole grain sandwich-type breads, rolls, and bagels
- Whole grain pita bread
- Low-fat bran or whole grain muffins
- Minimally processed cereals such as oatmeal, steel-cut oats, raisin bran, shredded wheat, and puffed wheat
- Boiled or steamed rice, barley, bulgur wheat and other whole grains
- Popcorn without butter
- Whole grain pasta

AGE-Less Tips for Breads, Cereals and Grains

- Toasting bread increases AGEs, but the amount is still a great deal less than the AGEs in meat or fat. For instance, one half of a bagel (1 ounce) contains about 30 kU AGE. Toasting increases the amount to about 50 kU. However, spread the bagel with just one teaspoon of butter and you add over 600 kU of AGEs!
- To satisfy a taste for grilled food, try a quesadilla filled with mashed black beans or grilled vegetables and low-fat cheese. Minimize AGE formation by coating the pan with a spritz of nonstick cooking spray instead of frying in butter, margarine, or oil.
- Substitute wedges of whole grain pita bread or thinly sliced bagel rounds for crackers.
- Garnish salads with canned chickpeas or kidney beans instead of browned or fried croutons.
- While grains (and starchy foods like potatoes) are low in AGEs, be careful not to overdo portions. Eating too much of a high-carb food at once can make blood sugar levels spike and increase AGE formation in the body.

Snack Foods and Sweets

Snack foods that are overly processed and contain added sugars and/ or fats, such as crackers, chips, pretzels, cookies, and pastries, can be quite high in AGEs. These same foods can also rocket blood sugar levels sky high, favoring the formation of AGEs in the body. So a tendency to rely on "grab-and-go" snack foods and to indulge in sugary sweets can spell double-trouble. The best advice is to think of snacks as mini-meals and snack on "real" food such as half a sandwich or a cup of soup instead of processed and sugary snacks. Here are some other lower-AGE ideas for snacks and sweets:

- Fresh fruit
- Yogurt (lower-sugar varieties)
- Low-fat mozzarella string cheese
- Hard-boiled egg
- Fresh vegetables with bean dip or low-fat dressing
- Whole grain cereal with milk
- Glass of milk and a low-fat bran muffin
- Mini whole grain bagel
- Low-fat popcorn
- Baked tortilla chips with salsa or bean dip
- Small piece of dark chocolate
- Pudding (low-sugar or sugar-free)
- Gelatin (sugar-free)
- Low-fat ice cream or frozen yogurt
- Sorbet
- Frozen fruit pop
- Frozen grapes

AGE-Less Tips for Snack Foods and Sweets

- Low-fat chips, crackers, and cookies tend to be lower in AGEs than high-fat versions, but can still contain significant amounts of AGEs (about 300-500 kU for just one ounce). Eat in moderation.

- Choose raw nuts and seeds rather than roasted or toasted ones.
- Choose lower-sugar and lower-calorie versions of sweets where possible. Keeping sugar levels down will help prevent AGEs from forming during digestion and in the bloodstream.
- Learn to be satisfied with just a few bites of a rich dessert.

Fats, Oils, Spreads and Dressings

Making smart fat choices is a high-priority of the AGE-Less Way. Fats and oils can contain high levels of AGEs, which form during refining and processing. One tablespoon of oil or margarine can contain over 500 kU AGE. Butter is several times higher. So it's key to avoid excess fat and choose less processed fats to stay within the range of 5,000 to 8,000 kU AGE daily. Choose these often to get your "good fats" with fewer AGEs:

- Nonfat and low-fat mayonnaise
- Salad dressings—Nonfat dressings are virtually AGE-free. "Light" dressings with no more than 5 to 6 grams fat per serving are also good choices. Go easy on sweet dressings to keep sugar under control.
- Margarine—Choose brands made from non-hydrogenated oils to minimize unhealthy trans-fats. Keep portions small and try "light" (which contain about 5 grams of fat per tablespoon) instead of full-fat versions (with 10 to 11 grams of fat per tablespoon).
- Olive oil—Choose cold-press "extra virgin" olive oil, which is the least refined and highest in AGE-fighting antioxidants and phytonutrients.
- Canola oil is a good source of healthy omega-3 fat, which helps to quench inflammation in the body. However, like all oils, it does contain AGEs, so use in moderation.
- Avocado—One ounce (about 1/4 cup cubed) contains about 500 kU AGE. However, since avocados are an unprocessed natural food, you also get important nutrients that make them a healthier fat choice than processed fats and oils. Use in moderation.
- Nuts and seeds—These foods do contain AGEs but are still con-sidered a healthy source of fat since they also provide beneficial

antioxidants, phytonutrients, fibers, and protein. Eating an ounce of nuts or seeds per day (3 to 4 tablespoons), *instead* of other fats, can protect against heart disease and diabetes. Be sure to choose raw nuts and seeds, since roasting increases their AGE content significantly.

AGE-Less Tips for the Fat Category

- Add a bit of healthy fat to salads and veggies for a more powerful antioxidant punch. Studies show that people who eat salads with light or regular dressing or some avocado slices absorb more beta-carotene, lycopene, and other antioxidants than people who use only nonfat dressing. A sprinkling of non-toasted nuts, ground flaxseed, chia, or olives would be expected to provide the same benefit. Just don't go overboard with fats since they do contain AGEs and are also high in calories.
- Stay away from roasted or toasted oils such as dark (toasted) sesame oil. The extra heat treatment greatly increases AGEs.
- Cook with fats that have a high smoke point, such as olive and canola oils. When fats smoke and turn brown, they are forming more AGEs. Avoid browning fats by all means!

Condiments and Seasonings

Use condiments and seasonings to perk up the flavor of foods, instead of age-accelerating AGEs. Choose from the following:

- Mustard
- Ketchup—Use in moderation due to high sugar content.
- Nonfat and light salad dressings—Try tossing vegetables with some light Italian or balsamic dressing before grilling or roasting or use as a marinade for meats to reduce AGE formation during cooking. Avoid brands that are high in sugar.
- Vinegar—Experiment with many different flavors including red wine, white wine, apple cider, rice, balsamic, raspberry, and more.

- Lemon juice
- Soy sauce
- Chili and hot peppers—If you like it hot and spicy, enjoy knowing that these seasonings are rich in AGE-defying antioxidants.
- Salsa
- Pickles
- Capers—These tiny brine- or salt-cured flower buds have long been used to perk up the flavor of pasta, seafood, chicken, and other Mediterranean fare. Capers are rich in antioxidants that neutralize oxidized fats in foods, making them a smart addition to your AGE-Less recipes. Keep in mind that capers are very salty, so be sure to cut back on salt elsewhere when adding them to your recipes.
- Herbs and spices (fresh or dried) are especially beneficial since they are loaded with antioxidants and phytonutrients that have their own anti-aging powers.
- Bouillon (vegetable, beef, or chicken)

Beverages

Many beverages are AGE-Less choices. Choose from the following:

- Coffee—Hold the sugar and lighten your coffee with milk instead of cream.
- Tea—Both green and black tea are rich in AGE-fighting antioxidants. Again, hold the sugar and lighten with milk instead of cream.
- Milk—All milk, even whole, is low in AGEs. Choose nonfat and low-fat versions for drinking to keep calories and saturated fats low. You may opt to use whole milk in coffee and recipes instead of cream.
- Diet sodas—Try to stay away from dark colored sodas (Part 1, Chapter 3). Their AGEs may add up if you drink large volumes.
- Tomato juice, vegetable juice
- Wine

PART 3:

Recipes and Strategies

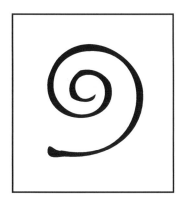

⊙ Chapter 11
Breakfast Recipes

Starting your day the AGE-Less Way can be a snap since many favorite breakfast foods are naturally low in AGEs. Whole grain breads and cereals, fruit, yogurt, milk, and eggs (especially the whites) are all good choices. Many AGE-Less breakfast options are so simple that no recipe is needed, which is perfect for busy weekday mornings. When you have a few minutes more, try these easy recipes for a tasty breakfast, brunch, or even a light dinner.

Poached Egg with Salmon & Tomato-Caper Salsa
Yield: 1 serving

1/2 ounce thinly sliced smoked salmon
1 poached egg
1 whole grain English muffin half, toasted

SALSA
1/4 cup chopped tomatoes
1 tablespoon chopped red onion
1 teaspoon finely chopped capers
1 1/2 teaspoons finely chopped fresh parsley

Combine all of the salsa ingredients in a small bowl and stir to mix. Set aside at room temperature for 20 to 30 minutes.

To assemble, place the English muffin half on a serving plate and top with the salmon, egg, and the salsa. Serve hot.

Nutritional Facts (per serving):

Calories: 175

Carbohydrates: 17 g

Fiber: 3 g

Fat: 6.8 g

Sat. Fat: 1.9 g

Cholesterol: 215 mg

Protein: 12 g

Sodium: 616 mg

Calcium: 122 mg

Diabetic exchanges: 1 starch, 1 1/2 medium-fat meat

Egg Quesadilla with Spinach & Cheese
Yield: 1 serving

2 tablespoons thinly sliced scallions or leeks
1/2 cup (packed) chopped fresh spinach
2 egg whites, beaten or 1/4 cup fat-free egg substitute
Freshly ground black pepper
1 whole wheat flour tortilla (8- to 9-inch round)
1/4 cup shredded reduced-fat mozzarella or Monterey Jack cheese
Olive oil cooking spray

Coat a large nonstick skillet with cooking spray and add the scallions or leeks. Cover and cook over medium heat for a couple of minutes to soften. Add the spinach and cook, covered, for another minute to wilt.

Distribute the vegetables evenly over the bottom of the skillet and pour the egg over the vegetables. Sprinkle with some pepper. Cover and cook, without stirring, for about a minute or until the eggs are set. Fold the eggs in half like an omelet.

Lay the tortilla out on a flat surface and place the egg over the bottom half of the tortilla. Sprinkle the cheese over the egg and fold the tortilla over to enclose the filling.

Respray the skillet and place over medium heat. Lay the filled tortilla in the skillet and spray the top lightly with the cooking spray.

Cook for about 1 1/2 minutes on each side or until nicely browned and the cheese is melted. Cut into wedges and serve hot.

Nutritional Facts (per serving):
Calories: 263
Carbohydrates: 29 g
Fiber: 2.6 g
Fat: 6.9 g
Sat Fat: 3.6 g
Cholesterol: 15 mg
Protein: 19 g
Sodium: 613 mg
Calcium: 333 mg
Diabetic Exchanges: 1 1/2 starch, 1 vegetable, 2 lean meat

Portabella Mushroom Omelet
Yield: 1 serving

3/4 cup sliced fresh baby portabella mushrooms
1/4 teaspoon herbs de Provence or fines herbs
Freshly ground black pepper
1/2 cup fat-free egg substitute or 2 egg whites, beaten
3 tablespoons shredded reduced-fat mozzarella cheese

Coat an 8-inch nonstick skillet with cooking spray and add the mushrooms and herbs. Sprinkle with pepper to taste. Cover and cook over medium heat for several minutes or until the mushrooms are tender and nicely browned. Remove and set aside to keep warm.

Respray the skillet and add the eggs. Cook without stirring for about a minute, or until set around the edges. Use a spatula to lift the edges of the omelet, and allow the uncooked egg to flow below the cooked portion. Cook for another minute, or until the eggs are almost set.

Scatter the mushrooms over one half of the omelet and sprinkle with the cheese. Fold the other half over the filling. Reduce the heat to low, cover and cook for about a minute, or until the cheese is melted and the eggs are set. Serve hot.

Nutritional Facts (per serving):
Calories: 127
Carbohydrate: 5 g
Fiber: 0.8 g
Fat: 3.5 g
Sat. Fat: 2.2 g
Cholesterol: 12 mg
Protein: 18 g
Sodium: 352 mg
Calcium: 181 mg
Diabetic exchanges: 3 lean meat

Caramelized Onion & Pepper Omelet
Yield: 1 serving

3/4 teaspoon extra virgin olive oil
1/3 medium yellow onion, very thinly sliced
4 thin slices red or green bell pepper, cut into half rings
1/4 teaspoon dried sage
1/8 teaspoon whole fennel seeds
1/8 teaspoon ground black pepper
1/2 cup fat-free egg substitute or 2 egg whites, beaten
1 tablespoon chopped fresh tomatoes
1 tablespoon crumbled reduced-fat feta cheese

Coat a small nonstick skillet with the olive oil. Add the onions, bell peppers, herbs, black pepper, and 2 teaspoons of water, and place over medium heat. Cover and cook for a couple of minutes, or until the vegetables start to soften. Reduce the heat to medium-low, and cook for about 5 minutes more, stirring occasionally, until the vegetables are soft and turn golden brown. (Add a little more water during cooking if the mixture becomes dry.) Transfer to a small dish and set aside to keep warm.

Wipe out and respray the skillet; preheat over medium heat. Add the eggs and reduce the heat to medium-low. Cook without stirring for a couple of minutes or until the eggs are set around the edges. Use a spatula to lift the edges of the omelet, and allow the uncooked egg to flow below the cooked portion. Cook for another minute or until the eggs are almost set.

Arrange the vegetables over half of the omelet. Fold the other half over the filling and cook for another minute or until the eggs are completely set. Slide the omelet onto a plate. Top with the tomatoes and feta. Serve hot.

Nutritional Facts (per serving):
Calories: 129
Carbohydrates: 8 g
Fiber: 1.4 g
Fat: 4.5 g
Sat. Fat: 1.1 g
Cholesterol: 2 mg
Protein: 14 g
Sodium: 351 mg
Calcium: 73 mg
Diabetic exchanges: 2 lean meat, 1 vegetable

Frittata Primavera
Yield: 2 servings

3/4 cup chopped fresh broccoli florets (1/2-inch pieces)
1/2 cup sliced fresh mushrooms
1/4 cup finely chopped red bell pepper
1/4 cup finely chopped yellow onion
1/2 teaspoon herbs de Provence or Italian seasoning
1/4 teaspoon ground black pepper
2 teaspoons extra virgin olive oil
1 teaspoon crushed garlic
1 cup fat-free egg substitute
1/3 cup shredded reduced-fat mozzarella cheese

Coat an 8-inch nonstick skillet with cooking spray. Add the vegetables, herbs, pepper, and 1 tablespoon of water. Cover and place over medium heat. Cook for several minutes, shaking the pan occasionally, until the vegetables are tender. Stir in the olive oil and garlic and cook for another 10 seconds.

Pour the egg substitute over the vegetables. Cover and cook without stirring for a couple of minutes, or until the edges start to set. Remove the lid and cook for a couple of minutes more, lifting the edges with a spatula, allowing uncooked egg to flow beneath the cooked portion, until the eggs are almost set.

Slide the frittata (wet side up) onto a large plate. Using potholders, place the skillet upside down over the frittata, and invert the frittata back into the skillet. Sprinkle with the cheese and reduce the heat to low. Cover and cook for about 30 seconds or just until the bottom is set. If the cheese has not melted, turn off the heat and let sit, covered, for another minute. Serve immediately.

Nutritional Facts (per serving):
Calories: 176
Carbohydrate: 8 g
Fiber: 2 g
Fat: 7.8 g Sat. Fat: 2.7 g
Cholesterol: 10 mg
Protein: 19 g
Sodium: 357 mg
Calcium: 196 mg
Diabetic exchanges: 2 1/2 lean meat, 1 vegetable, 1 fat

Spinach & Potato Frittata
Yield: 2 servings

3/4 cup cooked unpeeled new potatoes or Yukon Gold potatoes (1/4-inch dice)
1/4 cup finely chopped yellow onion
3/4 teaspoon herbs de Provence or fines herbs
1/4 teaspoon ground black pepper

2 teaspoons extra virgin olive oil
1 teaspoon crushed garlic
1 cup fat-free egg substitute
1 cup (packed) chopped fresh spinach
1/3 cup shredded reduced-fat mozzarella cheese

Coat an 8-inch nonstick skillet with cooking spray and add the potatoes, onion, herbs, pepper and 1 tablespoon of water. Cover and cook over medium heat for several minutes, shaking the pan occasionally, until the onion is tender and the potatoes are just beginning to brown. Add the olive oil and garlic; cover and cook for another 10 seconds. Toss in the spinach and cook and cover for another minute or until the spinach is wilted.

Spread the vegetables over the bottom of the skillet. Pour the eggs over the vegetables. Cover and cook without stirring, for a couple of minutes, or until set around the edges. Remove the lid and cook for a couple of minutes more, lifting the edges with a spatula, allowing the uncooked egg to flow beneath the cooked portion, until the frittata is almost set.

Slide the frittata (wet side up) onto a large plate. Using potholders, place the skillet upside down over the frittata, and invert the frittata back into the skillet. Sprinkle the cheese over the top. Cover and cook for about 30 seconds or just until the bottom of the frittata is set. If the cheese has not melted, turn off the heat and let sit, covered, for another minute. Cut in half and serve hot.

Nutritional Facts (per serving):
Calories: 198
Carbohydrate: 14 g
Fiber: 1.8 g
Fat: 7.8 g
Sat. Fat: 2.6 g
Cholesterol: 10 mg
Protein: 19 g
Sodium: 361 mg

Calcium: 202 mg
Diabetic exchanges: 2 1/2 lean meat, 1 carbohydrate

Cauliflower & Feta Cheese Frittata
Yield: 2 servings

1 1/2 cups fresh cauliflower florets (about 1/2-inch pieces)
1/4 cup water
1 1/2 teaspoons extra virgin olive oil
1/2 teaspoon crushed garlic
1 cup fat-free egg substitute
Freshly ground black pepper
2 tablespoons crumbled reduced-fat feta cheese with sun-dried tomatoes and herbs
2 tablespoons finely chopped fresh parsley

Coat an 8-inch nonstick skillet with cooking spray. Add the cauliflower and water and place over medium heat. Cover and cook for about 5 minutes or until the cauliflower is tender. If there is any excess liquid in the skillet, drain it off. Stir in the olive oil and garlic and cover for an additional 30 seconds.

Pour the eggs over the cauliflower mixture and sprinkle with some black pepper. Cook without stirring, for a minute or two or until the edges start to set. Continue to cook for a few minutes more, lifting the edges with a spatula, allowing uncooked egg to flow beneath the cooked portion, until the frittata is almost set.

Slide the frittata onto a large plate (wet side up). Using potholders, place the skillet upside down over the frittata, and invert the frittata back into the skillet. Cook for another minute or just until the bottom of the frittata is set. Cut the frittata in half and serve hot, topping each serving with a sprinkling of feta cheese and parsley.

Nutritional Facts (per serving):
Calories: 137
Carbohydrate: 7 g
Fiber: 2 g
Fat: 4.3 g
Sat. Fat: 1 g
Cholesterol: 2 mg
Protein: 18 g
Sodium: 430 mg
Calcium: 84 mg
Diabetic exchanges: 2 1/2 lean meat, 1 vegetable

Egg & Potato Skillet
Yield: 4 servings

1/3 cup chopped yellow onion
1/3 cup chopped green bell pepper
1/3 cup chopped red bell pepper
1/4 teaspoon sea salt
1/4 teaspoon ground black pepper
1/2 cup reduced-sodium vegetable or chicken broth (approximately)
2 2/3 cups cooked unpeeled Yukon Gold potatoes (1/4-inch dice)
4 large eggs
1/2 cup shredded reduced-fat cheddar cheese

Coat a medium-large nonstick skillet with cooking spray and add the onion, bell peppers, salt, and black pepper. Add 2 tablespoons of the broth; cover and cook over medium heat for several minutes or until tender. Add a little more broth if necessary to prevent scorching.

Add the potatoes and 3 tablespoons of the broth to the skillet and stir to mix. Cover and cook over medium heat for several minutes, stirring occasionally, until lightly browned. Shove the potatoes to one side of the skillet and re-spray the bottom. Redistribute the potatoes to cover the bottom of the skillet.

Make 4 small wells in the potato mixture. Crack the eggs and place 1 egg in each well. Reduce the heat to medium-low and drizzle 2 tablespoons of the broth over the skillet mixture. Cover and cook for 3 minutes or until the eggs are almost done.

Reduce the heat to low and sprinkle the cheese over the top. Cover and cook for 1 minute or until the cheese is melted and the eggs are done. Use a spatula to divide the mixture into 4 servings and transfer to serving plates. Serve hot.

Nutritional Facts (per serving)
Calories: 185
Carbohydrates: 20 g
Fiber: 2.6 g
Fat: 7.3 g
Sat. Fat: 3 g
Cholesterol: 219 mg
Protein: 13 g
Sodium: 423 mg
Calcium: 142 mg
Diabetic exchanges: 1 starch, 1 1/2 medium-fat meat

Southwestern-Style Eggs
Yield: 4 servings

1 cup canned black beans in seasoned sauce, non-drained and mashed with a fork
4 corn tortillas
4 large steam-basted or poached eggs (see page 137)
1/4 cup salsa
1/4 cup shredded reduced-fat Mexican blend or cheddar cheese
1/4 cup sliced scallions

Place the beans in a small pot. Cover and cook over medium heat for a minute or two to heat through. Set aside to keep warm.

Preheat an ungreased nonstick skillet over medium heat. Heat each tortilla in the skillet for about 15 seconds on each side. Place a tortilla on each of 4 serving plates. Spread one quarter of the beans over each tortilla and top with an egg and one quarter of the salsa, cheese, and scallions. Serve hot.

Nutritional Facts (per serving):
Calories: 215
Carbohydrates: 25 g
Fiber: 5.5 g
Fat: 7 g
Sat. Fat: 2.4 g
Cholesterol: 216 mg
Protein: 14 g
Sodium: 365 mg
Calcium: 136 mg
Diabetic exchanges: 2 lean meat, 1 1/2 starch

Sausage & Egg Burrito
Yield: 1 serving

1 vegetarian sausage link (1 ounce)
1/4 cup fat-free egg substitute or 1 large egg, beaten
1 whole wheat flour tortilla (8-inch round)
2 tablespoons shredded reduced-fat Mexican blend or cheddar cheese
1 tablespoon salsa (optional)

Coat a small nonstick skillet with cooking spray; add the sausage and 1 tablespoon water. Cover and cook over medium heat for a couple of minutes to heat through. Chop with a spatula to crumble and cook and cover for another minute.

Add the egg to the skillet and reduce the heat to medium-low. Cook, stirring slowly with a spatula, for about a minute to scramble.

Lay the tortilla on a flat surface and place the egg on the lower half, stopping about 1 inch from the bottom and sides. Sprinkle with the cheese and top with the salsa, if using. Fold in the sides and roll up from the bottom to enclose the filling. Cut in half and serve hot.

Nutritional Facts (per serving):
Calories: 265
Carbohydrates: 29 g
Fiber: 3.5 g
Fat: 6.5 g
Sat Fat: 2.4 g
Cholesterol: 8 mg
Protein: 21 g
Sodium: 751 mg
Calcium: 220 mg
Diabetic Exchanges: 2 starch, 2 1/2 lean meat

Apricot-Almond Muesli
Yield: 1 serving

3/4 cup light vanilla yogurt
1/4 cup plus 2 tablespoons old-fashioned oats
1/2 cup diced fresh apricots or canned (drained) apricots in natural juice,
or 2 tablespoons chopped dried apricots
1 tablespoon raw (non-toasted) wheat germ
1 tablespoon sliced almonds

Place all of the ingredients in a bowl and stir to mix. Let sit for 10 to 15 minutes before serving.

Nutritional Facts (per serving)
Calories: 324
Carbohydrates: 53 g
Fiber: 6 g
Fat: 5.2 g
Sat. Fat: 0.6 g
Cholesterol: 0 mg
Protein: 17 g

Sodium: 156 mg

Calcium: 384 mg

Diabetic exchanges: 1 starch, 1 fruit, 1 milk, 1 fat

For variety: Substitute fresh or canned peaches or pears for the apricots and pecans or walnuts for the almonds.

Hot & Hearty Oats
Yield: 3 servings

3/4 cup steel-cut oats
1/2 cup wheat bran
3 cups water (or use half water and half nonfat or low-fat milk)
1/4 cup raw (non-toasted) wheat germ

Place the oats, wheat bran, and water in a 3-quart pot and bring to a boil. Reduce the heat to maintain a simmer; cover and cook for 20 to 40 minutes (depending on the thickness of the oats), until the oats are tender. Stir occasionally to prevent the pot from boiling over.

Stir in the wheat germ. Remove from the heat and let sit covered for 5 minutes. Serve hot, with milk and/or fruit toppings if desired.

Nutritional Facts (per 1 1/8 cup-serving):

Calories: 225

Carbohydrates: 40 g

Fiber: 10.4 g

Fat: 4.3 g

Sat. Fat: 0.7 g

Cholesterol: 0 mg

Protein: 9.7 g

Sodium: 1 mg

Calcium: 31 mg

Diabetic exchanges: 2 1/2 starch

Hot Buckwheat Cereal with Apples & Walnuts
Yield: 4 servings

1/2 cup uncooked brown rice
1/2 cup uncooked roasted buckwheat (kasha)
2 cups water
2 cups nonfat or low-fat milk
1 cup canned no-added-sugar apple pie filling, chopped or Steamed Apples
(see page 271)
1/4 cup raisins
1/3 cup chopped walnuts

Place the rice in a blender and process for about 30 seconds, or until the texture of coarse grits.

Place the rice, buckwheat, water, and milk in a 2 1/2-quart non-stick pot and bring to a boil. Reduce the heat to maintain a simmer and keep cooking with the cover on for about 20 minutes, stirring every few minutes, until the mixture is thick and the grains are tender. Remove from the heat and let sit, covered for 5 minutes before serving.

Serve hot, topping each serving with some of the apples, raisins, and walnuts.

Nutritional Facts (per serving):
Calories: 316
Carbohydrates: 53 g
Fiber: 3.9 g
Fat: 7.4 g
Sat. Fat: 0.8 g
Cholesterol: 2 mg
Protein: 11.6 g
Sodium: 80 mg
Calcium: 173 mg
Diabetic exchanges: 2 starch, 1/2 nonfat/low-fat milk, 1 fruit, 1 fat

Quinoa with Bananas, Raisins & Pecans
Yield: 4 servings

1 cup uncooked quinoa
1 1/2 cups nonfat or low-fat milk
1 1/2 cups water
1/4 cup plus 2 tablespoons golden raisins
1 medium banana, sliced
1/4 cup chopped pecans

Place the quinoa in a wire strainer and rinse well with cool running water. Drain, place in a 2 1/2-quart pot, and add the milk and water. Bring to a boil and then reduce the heat to maintain a simmer. Cover and cook, stirring occasionally, for 20 minutes or until the quinoa is tender and most of the liquid is absorbed.

Add the raisins and simmer for 5 more minutes with the cover on. Stir in a little more milk if needed. Remove from the heat and let sit covered for 5 minutes. Stir in the bananas and pecans. Serve hot with low-calorie sweetener or a drizzle of honey if desired.

Nutritional Facts (per 1 1/8-cup serving):
Calories: 310
Carbohydrates: 52 g
Fiber: 4.5 g
Fat: 8.2 g
Sat. Fat: 0.9 g
Cholesterol: 2 mg
Protein: 10 g
Sodium: 59 mg
Calcium: 153 mg
Diabetic exchanges: 2 starch, 1 fruit, 1/2 nonfat/low-fat milk, 1 fat

Buttermilk French Toast
Yield: 6 slices

1/2 cup fat-free egg substitute
1/2 cup nonfat or low-fat buttermilk
1/4 teaspoon vanilla extract
1/8 teaspoon ground cinnamon
6 slices whole grain bread (1 ounce each)

Combine the egg substitute, buttermilk, vanilla, and cinnamon in a shallow bowl and whisk to mix. Dip the bread into the egg mixture, soaking both sides.

Coat a large nonstick skillet or griddle with cooking spray and preheat over medium heat until a drop of water sizzles when added. Cook the bread slices for about 1 1/2 minutes on each side or until light golden brown. Serve immediately. Top with warm canned no-added-sugar apple or cherry pie filling or Warm Strawberry Sauce (see page 133) if desired.

Nutritional Facts (per slice):
Calories: 89
Carbohydrate: 14 g
Fiber: 2 g
Fat: 1.3 g
Sat. Fat: 0.3 g
Cholesterol: 1 mg
Protein: 5.5 g
Sodium: 201 mg
Calcium: 56 mg
Diabetic exchanges: 1 starch

Filled Pancakes with Fruit Sauce
Yield: 4 servings

1/2 cup whole-wheat pastry flour
1/2 cup oat bran

1 tablespoon sugar
2 teaspoons baking powder
1 1/4 cups nonfat or low-fat buttermilk
3/4 cup fat-free egg substitute or 3 large eggs, beaten
1 cup nonfat or low-fat Greek-style yogurt
1 1/3 cups canned no-added-sugar cherry or apple pie filling or Warm Strawberry Sauce (see page 133)

Place the flour, oat bran, sugar, and baking powder in a medium bowl and stir to mix. Add the buttermilk and egg substitute or eggs and whisk until smooth. Set the batter aside for 5 minutes and whisk again.

Coat a large griddle or skillet with cooking spray and preheat over medium heat until a drop of water sizzles when it hits the heated surface. For each pancake, pour 1/3 cup of batter onto the griddle and use a spoon to spread it into a 6-inch circle. Cook for about 1 1/2 minutes or until the top is bubbly and the edges are dry. Turn and cook for about 30 seconds more, or until the second side is lightly browned. Repeat with the remaining batter to make 8 pancakes.

As the pancakes are done, spread 2 tablespoons of yogurt along one side. Roll up the pancake to enclose the filling and set aside to keep warm. To serve, place two roll-ups on each of 4 serving plates and top each serving with 1/3 cup of the pie filling or sauce. Serve warm.

Nutritional Facts (per serving):
Calories: 181
Carbohydrates: 34 g
Fiber: 4.2 g
Fat: 1.1 g
Sat. Fat: 0.2 g
Cholesterol: 0 mg
Protein: 13 g
Sodium: 366 mg
Calcium: 190 mg
Diabetic exchanges: 2 carbohydrate, 1 lean meat

Whole Grain Hot Cakes
Yield: 12 pancakes

1/2 cup quick-cooking (1-minute) oats
1 1/2 cups nonfat or low-fat buttermilk
1 cup whole wheat pastry flour or spelt flour
1 tablespoon sugar
2 teaspoons baking powder
1/2 cup fat-free egg substitute

Place the oats and buttermilk in a medium bowl and stir to mix. Set aside for 5 minutes. Place the flour, sugar, and baking powder in a small bowl and stir to mix. Set aside. Stir the egg substitute into the oat mixture. Add the flour mixture to the oat mixture and stir to mix.

Coat a large nonstick skillet or griddle with cooking spray and preheat over medium heat until a drop of water sizzles when added. For each pancake, pour 1/4 cup of batter onto the griddle or skillet and spread into a 4-inch circle. Cook for about 1 1/2 minutes, or until the top is bubbly and the edges are dry. Turn and cook for an additional minute, or until the second side is light golden brown.

Serve hot. If desired, top each serving with warm low-sugar apple pie filling, low-sugar jam, or Warm Strawberry Sauce (see page 133).

Nutritional Facts (per pancake):
Calories: 71
Carbohydrates: 13 g
Cholesterol: 1 mg
Fat: 0.7 g
Sat. Fat: 0.2 g
Fiber: 1.7 g
Protein: 3.9 g
Sodium: 134 mg
Calcium: 86 mg
Diabetic exchanges: 1 starch

Warm Strawberry Sauce
Yield: about 2 1/4 cups

3 cups chopped fresh or frozen (unthawed) strawberries (or substitute frozen mixed berries)
1/4 cup plus 2 tablespoon orange juice
Sugar substitute equal to 1/4 cup sugar
2 tablespoons sugar
1/4 cup water
1 tablespoon cornstarch

Place the strawberries, juice, sugar substitute, sugar, and half of the water in a 2-quart pot and place over medium heat. Cover and cook, stirring occasionally for 6 to 8 minutes, until the mixture comes to a boil and the berries soften and begin to break down.

Combine the remaining water and the cornstarch and stir to dissolve the cornstarch. Stir into the hot berry mixture. Cook and stir for another minute or until thickened and bubbly. Serve warm over French toast or pancakes.

Nutritional Facts (per 1/4-cup serving):
Calories: 38
Carbohydrates: 9 g
Fiber: 1.3 g
Fat: 0.2 g
Sat. Fat: 0 g
Cholesterol: 0 mg
Protein: 0.4 g
Sodium: 1 mg
Calcium: 9 mg
Diabetic exchanges: 1/2 carbohydrate

Cocoa-Banana Muffins
Yield: 12 muffins

1 1/2 cups oat bran
1/2 cup cocoa powder
1/2 cup brown sugar
1 teaspoon baking powder
1/4 teaspoon baking soda
1/4 teaspoon ground cinnamon
3/4 cup nonfat or low-fat milk
3/4 cup mashed very ripe banana
1/4 cup fat-free egg substitute or 1 large egg, beaten
2 tablespoons canola oil
1/3 cup chopped walnuts, almonds, or pecans
1/3 cup raisins (optional)

Preheat the oven to 350 degrees F. Combine the oat bran, cocoa powder, sugar, baking powder, baking soda, and cinnamon in a medium bowl and stir to mix. Combine the milk, banana, egg substitute or egg, and oil and stir to mix. Add the milk mixture to the oat bran mixture and stir to mix. Set the batter aside for 10 minutes and then stir in the nuts and raisins (if using).

Coat muffin cups with cooking spray, and divide the batter among the cups. Bake for about 15 minutes, or just until a wooden toothpick inserted in the center of a muffin comes out clean.

Remove the muffins from the oven, and let sit for 5 minutes before removing from the pan. Cool on wire racks and store in an airtight container. Refrigerate or freeze leftovers not eaten within 24 hours.

Nutritional Facts (per muffin):
Calories: 139
Carbohydrates: 23 g
Fiber: 3.3 g
Fat: 5.5 g
Sat. fat: 0.7 g

Cholesterol: 0 mg

Protein: 4.9 g

Sodium: 91 mg

Calcium: 66 mg

Diabetic exchanges: 1 1/2 carbohydrate, 1 fat

Apple Bran Muffins
Yield: 12 muffins

1 1/3 cups wheat bran
1 cup whole wheat pastry flour
1/4 cup dark brown sugar
1 1/4 teaspoons baking powder
1/4 teaspoon baking soda
1 cup nonfat or low-fat milk
1/4 cup honey or molasses
1/4 cup fat-free egg substitute or 1 large, egg beaten
2 tablespoons canola oil
1 cup chopped apples (about 1/4-inch dice)
1/3 cup dark raisins
1/3 cup chopped walnuts (optional)

Preheat the oven to 350 degrees F. Place the wheat bran, flour, brown sugar, baking powder, and baking soda in a medium bowl, and stir to mix. Press out the lumps in the brown sugar.

Combine and mix the milk, molasses, egg substitute or egg, and oil. Add the milk mixture, apples, and raisins to the bran mixture, and stir to mix. Set the batter aside for 10 minutes. Stir the batter for about 5 seconds, adding the walnuts (if using).

Coat muffin cups with cooking spray, and divide the batter among the cups. Bake for about 16 minutes, or just until a wooden toothpick inserted in the center of a muffin comes out clean. Remove the muffins from the oven, and let sit for 5 minutes before removing from the pan. Cool on wire racks and store in an airtight container. Refrigerate or freeze leftovers not eaten within 24 hours.

Nutritional Facts (per muffin):

Calories: 132

Carbohydrates: 27 g

Fiber: 4.4 g

Fat: 2.8 g

Sat. fat: 0.2 g

Cholesterol: 0 mg

Protein: 3.6 g

Sodium: 104 mg

Calcium: 79 mg

Diabetic exchanges: 1 1/2 carbohydrate, 1/2 fat

Mocha-Banana Smoothie
Yield: 1 serving

1 cup nonfat or low-fat milk
1/2 cup frozen sliced bananas
1 tablespoon sugar-free instant chocolate pudding mix
Sugar substitute equal to 1 tablespoon sugar
1/2 teaspoon instant coffee granules
1 pinch ground cinnamon

Place all of the ingredients in a blender and process until smooth. Pour into a tall glass and serve immediately.

Nutritional Facts (per serving):

Calories: 180

Carbohydrates: 35 g

Fiber: 2 g

Fat: 0.8 g

Sat Fat: 0.4 g

Cholesterol: 5 mg

Protein: 9 g

Sodium: 292 mg

Calcium: 306 mg

Diabetic Exchanges: I nonfat/low-fat milk, I fruit

EGGS—AGE-LESS STYLE

Eggs are naturally low in AGEs. Keep them low by using one of these AGE-Less cooking methods. Keep in mind that the whites are lower in AGEs than the yolks and are also fat- and cholesterol-free. For recipes such as omelets and frittatas, consider using more whites and fewer yolks or a fat-free egg substitute.

Scrambled: For each serving, beat together 2 eggs plus 2 tablespoons milk (or use 1/2 cup fat-free egg substitute and omit the milk). Coat a skillet with cooking spray and place over medium heat until just hot enough to sizzle a drop of water. Add the eggs to the skillet and let cook for a minute or until they begin to set around the edges. Gently draw a spatula or wooden spoon across the bottom and sides of the pan, forming large curds.

Steam-basted: (a low-fat alternative to fried eggs): Coat a nonstick skillet with cooking spray and preheat over medium heat until a drop of water sizzles when added. Use a large skillet for 4 eggs or a medium skillet for 2 eggs. Break the eggs and slip into the pan. Immediately reduce the heat to medium-low and add 1 teaspoon of water per egg. Place a lid on the pan to hold in the steam. Cook for a couple of minutes, until the whites are set and the yolks thicken.

Poached: Fill a pot or deep skillet with 3 inches of water. Add 2 table-spoons of vinegar or lemon juice per quart of water. Bring the liquid to a boil. Reduce the heat to keep the water gently simmering. Break eggs, one at a time, into a custard cup. Hold the cup close to the water's surface and slip the eggs, one at a time into the water. Cook until the whites are set and the yolks thicken, about 3 to 5 minutes. Use a slotted spoon to lift out the eggs.

Hard-boiled: Place eggs in a single layer in a pot. Add enough water to cover the eggs by at least 1 inch. Cover the pot, bring to a boil and the turn off the heat. Let the eggs stand covered for 15 minutes for large sized eggs.

Food safety tip: Note that food safety guidelines recommend cooking eggs until both the yolk and the white are firm. Scrambled eggs should not be runny.

⊚ Chapter 12
Comforting Soups and Stews

It's hard to beat a steaming bowl of soup or stew for a versatile, economical, and comforting meal. You can now add AGE-Less to this list of attributes. Simmering meats, poultry, and seafood in a savory broth is an ideal moist-heat cooking method—which makes soups and stews a natural for AGE-Less dining. Soups and stews can create the perfect balance of ingredients for AGE-Less meal planning—moderate portions of lean protein combined with generous amounts of nutrient-packed vegetables, legumes, whole grains, and flavorful herbs and spices. Whether you are looking for a cup of soup to pair with a sandwich or salad, or a hearty stew for a one-dish meal, you will find plenty of ideas here that are perfect for your AGE-Less Way.

Savory Lentil Soup
Yield: about 6 1/2 cups

1 1/4 cups dried brown lentils (about 8 ounces)
1 medium yellow onion, cut into thin wedges
2 tablespoons extra virgin olive oil
1 1/2 teaspoons crushed garlic
3 bay leaves
4 1/2 cups water or unsalted vegetable broth
1/2 teaspoon sea salt
1/2 teaspoon ground black pepper
14 1/2-oz can diced tomatoes with green pepper, celery, and onion, crushed and not drained

Place the lentils, onion, olive oil, garlic, bay leaves, water or broth, salt, and pepper in a 4-quart pot and bring to a boil. Reduce the heat to maintain a simmer. Cover and cook for 35 minutes, until the lentils are tender.

Add the tomatoes and bring to a boil. Reduce the heat to a simmer and cook and cover for about 40 minutes more or until the lentils are soft and the liquid is thick. Add a little more water if needed during cooking. If desired, drizzle each serving with a little red wine vinegar and olive oil.

Nutritional Facts (per 1-cup serving):
Calories: 172
Carbohydrates: 25 g
Fiber: 9 g
Fat: 4.5 g
Sat. Fat: 0.6 g
Cholesterol: 0 mg
Protein: 9 g
Sodium: 319 mg
Calcium: 43 mg
Diabetic exchanges: 1 lean meat, 1 carbohydrate, 1 fat

Fasolada (Greek White Bean Soup)
Yield: about 6 1/2 cups

1 1/4 cups dried white beans, such as navy or great northern (about 8 ounces), soaked and drained
2 medium yellow onions, cut into thin wedges
1 1/2 cups diced carrots
1 cup thinly sliced celery
4 cups water
2 teaspoons vegetable or chicken bouillon granules
1/2 teaspoon ground black pepper
2 tablespoons extra virgin olive oil
1/2 teaspoon sea salt

2 tablespoons finely chopped fresh parsley
Fresh lemon juice

Place the beans in a 4-quart pot and add the onion, carrots, celery, water, bouillon, pepper, and 1 tablespoon of the olive oil. Cover the pot and bring to a boil. Reduce the heat to low and simmer for 1 1/2 hours or until the beans are soft and the liquid is thick. Add a little more water during cooking if needed.

Stir in the salt, parsley, and the remaining olive oil. Cover and let sit for 5 minutes. Serve hot, adding a little lemon juice (about 1/2 teaspoon per cup) to each serving.

Nutritional Facts (per 1-cup serving):
Calories: 180
Carbohydrates: 28 g
Fiber: 6.9 g
Fat: 4.8 g
Sat. Fat: 0.8 g
Cholesterol: 0 mg
Protein: 8 g
Sodium: 466 mg
Calcium: 79 mg
Diabetic exchanges: 1 1/2 carbohydrate, 1 lean meat, 1/2 fat

Harvest Black Bean Chili
Yield: about 7 cups

1 tablespoon olive oil
1 cup chopped yellow onion
1 1/2 teaspoons crushed garlic
1 1/2 cups peeled cubed butternut squash (1/2-inch dice)
1 cup unsalted vegetable or chicken broth
1 1/2 tablespoons chili powder
1 teaspoon ground cumin

14 1/2-ounce can of no-salt diced tomatoes with peppers and onion, crushed and not drained
2 cans (15-ounces each) black beans, not drained
3/4 cup plus 2 tablespoons shredded reduced-fat Monterey Jack or white cheddar cheese

Add the olive oil, onion, and 1 tablespoon of water to a 4-quart pot. Cover and cook over medium heat for several minutes until the onion starts to soften. Add the garlic and cook for another 30 seconds.

Add the squash, broth, chili powder, and cumin and bring to a boil. Cover and cook over medium heat for about 8 minutes, or until almost tender. Add the tomatoes and black beans and adjust the heat to maintain a simmer. Cover and cook for about 10 minutes, until the squash is tender. Serve hot, topping each serving with a sprinkling of cheese.

Nutritional Facts (per 1-cup chili with 2 tablespoons cheese):
Calories: 205
Carbohydrates: 26 g
Fiber: 9.6 g
Fat: 5.5 g
Sat. Fat: 1.8 g
Cholesterol: 7 mg
Protein: 13 g
Sodium: 509 mg
Calcium: 186 mg
Diabetic exchanges: 1 1/2 carbohydrate, 1 1/2 lean meat

Fiesta Chili
Yield: about 9 cups

1 pound ground beef (at least 93% lean)
1 cup chopped yellow onion
14 1/2-ounce can diced tomatoes with green chilies, do not drain
8-ounce can tomato sauce

3/4 cup beer (light or regular)
3 tablespoons chili powder
3/4 teaspoon dried oregano
2 cans (15 ounces each) dark red kidney beans, drained (reserve about 1/2 cup of the juice)
1 1/4 cups fresh or frozen whole kernel corn

Coat a 4-quart pot with cooking spray and add the ground beef and onion. Use a spatula to crumble the meat. Cover and cook over medium heat for about 6 minutes, stirring occasionally until the meat is no longer pink (do not drain).

   Add the tomatoes, tomato sauce, beer, chili powder, and oregano and bring to a boil. Reduce the heat to maintain a simmer. Cover and simmer for 15 minutes, stirring occasionally. Stir in the beans and corn and simmer covered for 15 minutes more. Add some of the reserved bean liquid if the mixture seems too thick. Serve hot.

Nutritional Facts (per 1-cup serving):
Calories: 238
Carbohydrates: 31 g
Fiber: 10.5 g
Fat: 4.6 g
Sat. Fat: 1.6 g
Cholesterol: 32 mg
Protein: 19 g
Sodium: 329 mg
Calcium: 26 mg
Diabetic exchanges: 2 lean meat, 1 1/2 carbohydrate

Beef Stew Provencal
Yield: 6 servings

1 1/2 pounds lean stew beef, cut into 1-inch chunks
14 1/2-ounce can of stewed tomatoes, not drained and pureed in a blender

1/2 cup dry red wine
1/2 cup water
1 tablespoon crushed garlic
2 teaspoons beef bouillon granules
1 1/2 teaspoons dried thyme
3/4 teaspoon dried rosemary
1/2 teaspoon ground black pepper
2 cups sliced fresh mushrooms
1 cup sliced carrot
2 yellow onions, cut into 1/2-inch wedges (about 2 cups)
3/4 cup frozen green peas
2 tablespoons whole wheat pastry flour or unbleached flour

Coat a 4-quart nonstick pot with cooking spray and preheat over medium heat. Add the beef and cook for a couple of minutes, just enough to lightly brown and seal the meat. Add the tomatoes, wine, water, garlic, bouillon, thyme, rosemary, and pepper and bring to a boil. Reduce the heat to maintain a simmer. Cover and cook for 45 minutes.

Add the mushrooms, carrot, and onions and return to a boil. Reduce the heat and simmer covered for 30 minutes or until meat and vegetables are tender. Add the peas and return to a simmer. Combine the flour and 2 tablespoons of water and whisk until smooth. Then, stir in 2 tablespoons of liquid from the pot into the flour mixture. Stir the flour mixture into the pot. Leave the pot uncovered and simmer, stirring occasionally, for 10 minutes.

Nutritional Facts (per 1 1/8-cup serving):
Calories: 265
Carbohydrates: 16 g
Fiber: 4 g
Fat: 7.9 g
Sat. Fat: 3.1 g
Cholesterol: 68 mg
Protein: 28 g
Sodium: 568 mg

Calcium: 40 mg

Diabetic exchanges: 3 lean meat, 1/2 starch, 2 vegetable

Beef & Barley Soup
Yield: 8 servings

3/4 pound ground beef (at least 93% lean)
2 cups sliced fresh mushrooms
3/4 cup chopped yellow onion (about 1 medium onion)
4 cups water
1 1/2 cups V-8 vegetable juice
1 cup (moderately packed) grated carrots
1/2 cup pearl barley
1 tablespoon beef bouillon granules
2 1/2 teaspoons crushed garlic
1 teaspoon dried thyme
1 bay leaf
1/2 teaspoon ground black pepper
2 tablespoons finely chopped fresh parsley or 2 teaspoons dried
2 teaspoons lemon juice

Coat a 4-quart nonstick pot with cooking spray. Add the ground beef, mushrooms, and onion and use a spatula to break up the meat. Place over medium heat; cover and cook, stirring to crumble, for about 5 minutes or until the meat is no longer pink (do not drain). Add the remaining ingredients except for the parsley and lemon juice and bring to a boil. Reduce the heat to maintain a simmer. Cover and cook for 45 to 50 minutes or until the barley is tender.

Remove the bay leaf and stir in the parsley. Let sit covered, for 3 minutes. Stir in the lemon juice and serve hot.

Nutritional Facts (per 1-cup serving):

Calories: 138

Carbohydrates: 16 g

Fiber: 3.1 g

Fat: 3.2 g
Sat. Fat: 1.3 g
Cholesterol: 27 mg
Protein: 11.2 g
Sodium: 471 mg
Calcium: 26 mg
Diabetic Exchanges: 1 1/2 lean meat, 1/2 starch, 1 vegetable

Meatball Soup
Yield: about 7 cups

4 cups water
1 1/4 cups V-8 vegetable juice
1/2 cup chopped carrot
1 tablespoon beef bouillon granules
2 teaspoons crushed garlic
1/4 teaspoon ground black pepper
4 ounces whole wheat orzo (about 2/3 cup)
4 cups (moderately packed) chopped fresh spinach
1/4 cup finely chopped fresh parsley or 4 teaspoons dried (garnish)

MEATBALLS
1/2 pound ground beef (at least 93% lean)
1/2 cup soft whole wheat bread crumbs*
1/4 cup finely chopped yellow onion
2 teaspoons dried parsley
1 teaspoon crushed garlic
1/4 teaspoon ground black pepper

Place all of the meatball ingredients in a large bowl and mix well. Shape into 21 meatballs (each slightly less than 1-inch diameter) and set aside.

Place the water, V-8 juice, carrot, bouillon, garlic, and pepper in a 4-quart pot. Cover and bring to a boil. Reduce the heat and simmer for 10 minutes. Use a stick blender to carefully blend the mixture until smooth. (Alternatively, use a slotted spoon to transfer the carrots to a blender, add about 1 1/2 cups of the broth and carefully blend at low speed until smooth. Pour the mixture back into the pot.)

Bring the pot to a boil over medium heat and add the meatballs. Cover and cook for 5 minutes, adjusting the heat to maintain a simmer. Add the orzo and simmer for 10 minutes or until almost tender. Add the spinach and cook for several minutes more, until the orzo is tender and the spinach is wilted. Add a little more V-8 juice or water if needed. Serve hot, topping each serving with a sprinkling of parsley.

Nutritional Facts (per 1-cup serving):
Calories: 136
Carbohydrates: 17 g
Fiber: 4 g
Fat: 2.8 g
Sat. Fat: 1 g
Cholesterol: 20 mg
Protein: 10 g
Sodium: 527 mg
Calcium: 50 mg
Diabetic exchanges: 1 lean meat, 1/2 starch, 1 vegetable

*Tear about 2/3 of a slice of whole wheat bread into pieces. Process into crumbs in a mini food processor.

Shrimp Gazpacho
Yield: 4 servings

2 cups chopped fresh tomatoes
1 1/2 cups diced peeled and seeded cucumber
1/2 cup chopped green bell pepper
1/2 cup chopped yellow bell pepper
1/2 cup chopped yellow or sweet white onion
2 teaspoons crushed garlic

3 tablespoons chopped fresh parsley
1 1/2 cups V-8 vegetable juice (regular or spicy)
2 tablespoons red wine vinegar
1 tablespoon plus 1 teaspoon extra virgin olive oil
3/4 teaspoon chili powder
1/4 teaspoon ground black pepper
1/4 teaspoon sea salt
2 1/2 cups boiled or steamed shrimp, chilled

Place the tomatoes, cucumber, bell peppers, onion, garlic, and 1 table-spoon of the parsley in the bowl of a food processor and process until chopped to a medium-fine texture. Place the chopped vegetables in a large bowl and add the vegetable juice, vinegar, olive oil, chili powder, black pepper, and salt. Add a little more vegetable juice if the mixture seems too thick.

Cover and chill for 1 to 5 hours before serving. Serve chilled, topping each serving with a quarter of the shrimp and a sprinkling of the remaining parsley.

Nutritional Facts (per serving):
Calories: 184
Carbohydrates: 14 g
Fiber: 3.3 g
Fat: 6 g
Sat. Fat: 0.9 g
Cholesterol: 161 mg
Protein: 20 g
Sodium: 587 mg
Calcium: 68 mg
Diabetic exchanges: 3 lean meat, 3 vegetable

Seafood Stew with Fire-Roasted Tomatoes
Yield: 4 servings

2 tablespoons extra virgin olive oil
1/2 cup plus 2 tablespoons finely chopped yellow onion
2 teaspoons crushed garlic
14 1/2-ounce can diced fire-roasted tomatoes, do not drain
1/2 cup dry white wine
1 tablespoon plus 1 teaspoon dried parsley
1/4 teaspoon crushed red pepper
1 dozen small (about 2-inches diameter) fresh clams in the shell
1/2 pound medium-size peeled and de-veined shrimp
1/2 pound scallops

Place half of the olive oil, 1 tablespoon of water, and all of the onion in a large, deep nonstick skillet. Cover and cook over medium heat for several minutes or until the onion softens. Add the garlic and cook for about 20 seconds more. Add the tomatoes, wine, parsley, and red pepper and bring to a boil. Cover and cook for 3 minutes.

Add the clams, cover and cook over medium-high heat for 3 minutes. Stir in the shrimp and scallops and continue to cover for 3 to 4 minutes more, or until the clamshells open and the shrimp and scallops turn opaque. Discard any clams that have not opened. Stir in the remaining olive oil and serve hot.

Nutritional Facts (per serving):
Calories: 260
Carbohydrates: 10 g
Fiber: 2.3 g
Fat: 8.9 g
Sat. Fat: 1.2 g
Cholesterol: 119 mg
Protein: 28 g
Sodium: 429 mg
Calcium: 109 mg
Diabetic exchanges: 3 1/2 lean meat, 1 vegetable, 1 fat

Chicken, Barley & Corn Chowder
Yield: about 8 cups

2 cups peeled and diced raw sweet potatoes or butternut squash
3/4 cup chopped yellow onion
5 cups water
1 1/2 tablespoons chicken bouillon granules
2 teaspoons crushed garlic
1 teaspoon dried marjoram
1/2 teaspoon dried thyme
1/4 teaspoon ground black pepper
1/2 cup uncooked pearl barley
2 bone-in skinless chicken breast halves (5 to 6 ounces each)
1 1/4 cups fresh or frozen whole kernel corn
2 tablespoons finely chopped fresh parsley or 2 teaspoons dried

Place the sweet potato or squash, onion, water, bouillon, garlic, marjoram, thyme, and pepper in a 4-quart pot and bring to a boil. Reduce the heat to maintain a simmer; cover and cook for about 10 minutes, or until the vegetables are soft. Use a stick blender to carefully blend the mixture until smooth. Stir for a minute or two to dissipate any foam that forms during blending.

Add the barley and chicken to the pot and bring to a boil. Reduce the heat to maintain a simmer; cover and cook for 40 minutes. Remove the chicken and set aside to cool slightly. Add the corn and cook for 10 minutes more, until the barley and corn are tender.

Remove the chicken from the bone and dice into small pieces. Add to the soup and simmer for a few minutes to heat through. Serve hot, topping each serving with a sprinkling of parsley.

Nutritional Facts (per 1-cup serving):
Calories: 158
Carbohydrates: 25 g
Fiber: 3.9 g

Fat: 1 g
Sat. Fat: 0.2 g
Cholesterol: 25 mg
Protein: 13 g
Sodium: 459 mg
Calcium: 23 mg
Diabetic exchanges: 1 1/2 lean meat, 1 1/2 starch

Chicken Tortilla Soup
Yield: 4 servings

1 medium yellow onion, cut into thin wedges (about 1 cup)
1/2 cup diced carrot
3 cups reduced-sodium chicken broth (or 3 cups water plus 1 1/2 teaspoons chicken bouillon)
2 boneless skinless chicken breast halves (4 ounces each)
14 1/2-ounce can of Mexican-style tomatoes, non-drained and pureed in a blender
3/4 teaspoon ground cumin
3/4 teaspoon dried oregano
1/4 teaspoon ground black pepper
1 cup fresh or frozen whole kernel corn
1 medium zucchini, quartered lengthwise and sliced (about 1 cup)

TORTILLA STRIPS
4 corn tortillas, cut into strips (about 1-by-1/2 inches)
Olive oil cooking spray
1/8 teaspoon sea salt (optional)

Place the onion, carrot, and 1/2 cup of the broth in a 4-quart pot and place over medium heat. Cover and cook for 5 minutes, until the vegetables start to soften. Add the chicken, remaining broth, pureed tomatoes, cumin, oregano, and pepper and bring to a boil. Reduce the heat to maintain a simmer and continue to cover for 20 minutes. Remove the chicken to a cutting board. Dice the meat and add it back to the pot.

Add the corn and cook for 10 minutes. Add the zucchini and cook for about another 5 minutes, or until the zucchini is tender.

While the soup is cooking, preheat the oven to 350 degrees F. Coat a baking sheet with cooking spray and arrange the strips in a single layer on the sheet. Spray the strips lightly with the cooking spray. If desired, sprinkle with the salt. Bake for about 8 to 10 minutes, or just until lightly browned and crisp. Serve the soup hot, topping each serving with some of the tortilla strips.

Nutritional Facts (per 1 1/2-cup serving plus tortilla strips):
Calories: 198
Carbohydrates: 31 g
Fiber: 5.1 g
Fat: 1.7 g
Sat. Fat: 0.3 g
Cholesterol: 33 mg
Protein: 18 g
Sodium: 725 mg
Calcium: 88 mg
Diabetic exchanges: 1 1/2 lean meat, 2 carbohydrate

Home-Style Chicken Soup
Yield: 6 servings

1 1/4 cups diced carrots
1/2 cup chopped onion
1/2 cup chopped celery
2 boneless skinless chicken breast halves (4 ounces each)
4 1/2 cups water
1 tablespoon plus 1 teaspoon chicken bouillon granules
2 teaspoons crushed garlic
Scant 1/4 teaspoon ground white pepper
2 1/2 ounces whole grain angel hair pasta, broken into 1-inch pieces (or substitute whole grain penne or rotini)

3/4 cup frozen green peas
1/4 to 1/3 cup finely chopped fresh parsley

Place the carrots, onion, celery, and chicken in a 4-quart pot. Add the water, bouillon, garlic, and pepper and bring to a boil. Reduce the heat to maintain a simmer. Cover and simmer for 20 minutes.

Remove the chicken to a cutting board and set aside. Use a slotted spoon to transfer about half of vegetables to a blender. Add about 1 1/2 cups of the broth and carefully blend at low speed until smooth. Pour the mixture back into the pot. Bring the soup to a boil and add the pasta. Reduce the heat to medium-low, cover and cook for about 5 minutes, stirring occasionally, until the pasta is almost tender. Dice the chicken and add it to the soup along with the peas. Cover and simmer for about 3 minutes more, or until the pasta is tender. Stir in the parsley and remove from heat. Let it sit covered for 3 minutes before serving.

Nutritional Facts (per 1-cup serving):
Calories: 114
Carbohydrates: 15 g
Fiber: 3.4 g
Fat: 0.8 g
Sat. Fat: 0.2 g
Cholesterol: 22 mg
Protein: 12 g
Sodium: 532 mg
Calcium: 30 mg
Diabetic Exchanges: 1 lean meat, 1 starch

Chunky Potato Soup
Yield: about 7 cups

1 1/4 cups chopped yellow onion
1 cup chopped celery

1 teaspoon crushed garlic
2 1/2 cups chicken or vegetable broth
2 cups diced carrots (slightly less than 1/2-inch pieces)
1/2 teaspoon sea salt
Scant 1/2 teaspoon ground black pepper
3 1/2 cups unpeeled Yukon Gold potatoes (slightly less than 1/2-inch dice)
1 1/2 cups whole milk
1 1/2 tablespoons finely chopped fresh dill or 1 1/2 teaspoons dried

Place the onion, celery, garlic, and 1/2 cup of the broth in a 4-quart nonstick pot. Cover and cook over medium heat for about 10 minutes, shaking the pan occasionally, until the vegetables are soft. Add a little water if needed to prevent scorching.

Add the carrots, remaining broth, salt, and pepper; bring to a boil. Cover and cook over medium heat for 5 minutes. Add the potatoes and return the pot to a boil. Cover and cook for about 15 minutes or until the potatoes and carrots are soft.

Place 2 1/2 cups of the vegetable mixture from the pot in a blender and add the milk. Carefully blend at low speed until pureed (use caution when blending hot liquids). Return the pureed mixture to the pot and cook for a few minutes to heat through. Add a little more milk if needed. Serve hot, topping each serving with a sprinkling of dill.

Nutritional Facts (per 1-cup serving):
Calories: 114
Carbohydrates: 23 g
Fiber: 3.4 g
Fat: 2.1 g
Sat. Fat: 1.1 g
Cholesterol: 7 mg
Protein: 4.5 g
Sodium: 522 mg

Calcium: 92 mg

Diabetic exchanges: 1 1/2 carbohydrate

Creamy Asparagus Soup
Yield: about 6 cups

2 teaspoons soft margarine or olive oil
1 cup chopped yellow onion
1/4 cup finely chopped celery
1 1/4 cups diced peeled Yukon Gold potato
2 cups chicken or vegetable broth
3/4 teaspoon dried fines herbes or thyme
1/4 teaspoon ground black pepper
5 cups 1-inch pieces fresh asparagus
1 cup whole milk

TOPPINGS
1/3 cup nonfat or light sour cream
2 tablespoons lemon juice
1 tablespoon finely chopped fresh dill (or 1 teaspoon dried)

Place the margarine or olive oil and 1 tablespoon of water in a 4-quart nonstick pot and place over medium heat. Add the onion and celery, cover and cook for several minutes, shaking the pan occasionally, until the vegetables start to soften. Add a few teaspoons of water if necessary to prevent scorching.

Add the potato, broth, fines herbes or thyme, and pepper to the pot. Cover, and bring to a boil. Reduce the heat to a simmer and cook for 5 minutes. Add the asparagus and return to a boil. Reduce the heat and simmer for about 6 to 8 minutes, until the potatoes and asparagus are soft. Use a stick blender to puree the mixture until smooth. (Alternatively, carefully puree the soup at low speed, 2 cups at a time, in a regular blender.) Stir in the milk and heat through, adding a little more milk if the mixture seems too thick.

Place the sour cream and lemon juice in a small bowl and whisk until smooth. Spoon the soup into bowls and drizzle some of the sour cream mixture over each serving. Top with a sprinkling of dill.

Nutritional Facts (per 1-cup serving):
Calories: 96
Carbohydrates: 14 g
Fiber: 2.6 g
Fat: 3 g
Sat. Fat: 1.1 g
Cholesterol: 5 mg
Protein: 4.5 g
Sodium: 327 mg
Calcium: 92 mg
Diabetic exchanges: 1/2 starch, 1 vegetable, 1/2 fat

Chapter 13: Sandwiches and Such

The humble sandwich is perhaps the all-time favorite fast-food solution. There are many reasons why sandwiches are perfect for the AGE-Less Way. For starters, most sandwich-type breads are quite low in AGEs. In addition, a wide range of savory fillings and spreads can be enjoyed on the AGE-Less Way. As a bonus, sandwiches are a great way to satisfy a taste for grilled or roasted foods since grilled and roasted breads and vegetables are quite low in AGEs compared to grilled or roasted meats. This section offers a bounty of hearty sandwiches and sandwich spin-offs such as quesadillas, pizzas, and wraps made the AGE-Less Way. Lower-AGE fillings such as poached chicken, tuna, eggs, and beans are combined with light spreads, lower-fat cheeses, plenty of colorful veggies, and whole grain breads to create an array of satisfying sandwiches. Pair your AGE-Less sandwich with a cup of soup or fruit for a tasty and filling meal anytime.

Bodacious Burgers
Yield: 4 servings

1 cup sliced fresh mushrooms
1 pound ground beef (at least 93% lean)
1 tablespoon Dijon or spicy mustard
1/2 teaspoon ground black pepper
4 whole grain burger buns
4 slices each of lettuce, tomato, and onion

Place the mushrooms in a food processor and process until very finely chopped. Transfer to a large bowl and add the ground meat, mustard, and pepper. Mix well and shape into 4 patties, each 4 inches in diameter. Shape the patties so that the centers are slightly thinner than the edges (to promote faster, more even cooking).

Coat a large nonstick skillet with cooking spray and place the burgers in the skillet. Cook for about 6 to 8 minutes, turning every couple of minutes, until the thickest part reaches 160 degrees F. Place a lid on the skillet, as needed, to maintain a couple of tablespoons of liquid in the skillet. Avoid pressing down on the burgers during cooking as this removes moisture. Serve the burgers in the buns with the lettuce, tomato, and onions. Add your choice of condiments.

Nutritional Facts (per serving):
Calories: 300
Carbohydrates: 26 g
Fiber: 4 g
Fat: 8.8 g
Sat. Fat: 3.2 g
Cholesterol: 70 mg
Protein: 30 g
Sodium: 371 mg
Calcium: 70 mg
Diabetic exchanges: 3 lean meat, 1 1/2 starch, 1 vegetable

Spicy Egg Salad Sandwiches
Yield: 4 servings

6 hard-boiled eggs, peeled and chopped
1/4 cup nonfat or light mayonnaise
1 tablespoon spicy mustard
1/2 cup finely chopped celery
1/4 cup thinly sliced scallions
1/4 cup chopped dill or sweet pickles, well drained
8 slices multigrain, dark rye, or pumpernickel bread (1.1 ounces each)
1 cup fresh arugula or watercress leaves

Place the eggs in a bowl and mash with a fork. Add the mayonnaise, mustard, celery, scallions, and pickles and stir to mix. Add a little more mayonnaise if needed. Top four of the bread slices with one-fourth of the egg salad and arugula or watercress leaves. Top with the remaining bread slices and cut each sandwich in half. Serve immediately.

Nutritional Facts (per serving):
Calories: 294
Carbohydrates: 35 g
Fiber: 4.6 g
Fat: 10.7 g
Sat. Fat: 3 g
Cholesterol: 318 mg
Protein: 16 g
Sodium: 743 mg
Calcium: 111 mg
Diabetic exchanges: 1 1/2 medium-fat meat, 2 starch

Mediterranean Tuna Wraps
Yield: 4 servings

3 cups mixed baby salad greens
6-ounce can of tuna in water, drained
3/4 cup marinated artichoke hearts, drained and chopped
1/2 cup shredded reduced-fat mozzarella cheese or 1/4 cup crumbled re-duced-fat feta cheese
2 slices red onion, cut into quarter-rings
2 tablespoons light olive oil vinaigrette salad dressing
4 whole-wheat flour tortillas (9-inch rounds)
8 slices plum tomato

Combine the salad greens, tuna, artichoke hearts, cheese, and onion in a large bowl. Drizzle the dressing over the mixture and toss to mix. Arrange one-fourth of the salad mixture over the bottom half of each tortilla, leaving a 1-inch margin on both sides. Top the salad mixture on each wrap with 2 slices of tomato. Fold in the sides and roll the tortillas up to enclose the filling. Cut in half and serve immediately.

Nutritional Facts (per serving):
Calories: 287
Carbohydrates: 32 g
Fiber: 5.2 g
Fat: 8.6 g
Sat. Fat: 2.2 g
Cholesterol: 20 mg
Protein: 21 g
Sodium: 647 mg
Calcium: 233 mg
Diabetic exchanges: 2 lean meat, 2 starch, 1 vegetable, 1/2 fat

Black Bean Quesadillas
Yield: 4 servings

1 cup canned black beans in seasoned sauce, drain off about 2/3 of the liquid and mash with a fork
2 to 4 teaspoons finely chopped pickled jalapeno peppers
4 whole wheat flour tortillas (8 to 9-inch rounds)
1 cup shredded reduced-fat mild cheddar or Monterey Jack cheese
Olive oil cooking spray

TOPPINGS
1/3 cup chopped tomatoes or salsa
1/3 cup nonfat or light sour cream
1/4 cup sliced scallions

Stir the jalapeno peppers into the mashed beans. Spread the bottom half of each tortilla with one-fourth of the beans and one-fourth of the cheese. Fold the top half of the tortillas over to enclose the filling.

Coat a large griddle or nonstick skillet with cooking spray, and preheat over medium heat until a drop of water sizzles when added.

Lay the quesadillas on the griddle and spray the tops lightly with the cooking spray. Cook for about 1 1/2 minutes on each side, or until nicely browned. Cut the quesadillas into wedges and serve hot, accompanied by the toppings.

Nutritional Facts (per serving):
Calories: 264
Carbohydrates: 38 g
Fiber: 6 g
Fat: 6.6 g
Sat. Fat: 3.5 g
Cholesterol: 15 mg
Protein: 15 g
Sodium: 680 mg
Calcium: 352 mg
Diabetic exchanges: 2 starch, 2 lean meat

Roasted Red Pepper Quesadillas
Yield: 4 servings

4 whole-wheat flour tortillas (8 to 9-inch rounds)
2/3 cup jarred roasted red bell pepper, well drained and chopped
1 tablespoon finely chopped fresh basil or 1 teaspoon dried basil
1 cup shredded reduced-fat mozzarella cheese
Olive oil cooking spray

Sprinkle the bottom half of each tortilla with one-fourth of the bell peppers, basil, and cheese. Fold the top half of the tortillas over to enclose the filling.

Coat a large griddle or nonstick skillet with cooking spray, and preheat over medium heat until a drop of water sizzles when added. Lay the quesadillas on the griddle and spray the tops lightly with the cooking spray. Cook for about 1 1/2 minutes on each side, or until nicely browned. Cut each quesadilla into wedges and serve hot.

Nutritional Facts (per serving):
Calories: 225
Carbohydrates: 27 g
Fiber: 2.4 g
Fat: 6.7 g
Sat. Fat: 3.6 g
Cholesterol: 15 mg
Protein: 12 g
Sodium: 489 mg
Calcium: 310 mg
Diabetic exchanges: 2 starch, 1 lean meat

Spinach Pita Pizzas
Yield: 4 servings

1/2 cup sliced scallions
2 cups chopped fresh spinach
3/4 teaspoon dried basil
3/4 teaspoon whole fennel seed
4 pieces whole grain pita bread (6-inch rounds)
1 cup low-fat marinara sauce
1 cup shredded part-skim mozzarella
Crushed red pepper (optional)

Preheat the oven to 400 degrees F. Coat a large nonstick skillet with cooking spray and add the scallions. Cover and cook over medium heat for a couple of minutes or until softened. Add the spinach and cook for another minute or two to wilt. Stir in the basil and fennel and set aside.

Place the pitas on a large baking sheet and spread each one with 1/4 cup of the marinara sauce. Top each pita with one-fourth of the spinach mixture. Bake for 8 minutes. Sprinkle the cheese over the pizzas and return to the oven. Turn off the oven and let the pizzas bake for 1 more minute, or just until the cheese is melted. Serve hot, topped with a sprinkling of crushed red pepper if desired.

Nutritional Facts:

Calories: 253

Carbohydrates: 39 g

Fiber: 5 g

Fat: 5.5 g

Sat. Fat: 3.1 g

Cholesterol: 15 mg

Protein: 16 g

Sodium: 598 mg

Calcium: 292 mg

Diabetic exchanges: 2 starch, 1 vegetable, 1 medium-fat meat

Very Veggie Sandwich
Yield: 1 serving

2 slices mixed grain or dark pumpernickel bread (1.1 ounces each)
1/4 cup Creamy Artichoke Spread (see page 259)
1 ounce thinly sliced reduced-fat mozzarella or Swiss cheese
1 slice red onion
4 slices cucumber
1 tablespoon grated carrot
4 fresh spinach leaves
1/3 cup alfalfa sprouts
1 1/2 teaspoons nonfat or light mayonnaise

Spread one bread slice with the artichoke spread. Top with the cheese, onion, cucumber, carrot, spinach, and sprouts. Spread the remaining bread slice with the mayonnaise and place on the sandwich. Cut in half and serve.

Nutritional Facts (per serving):

Calories: 319

Carbohydrates: 43 g

Fiber: 8 g

Fat: 8.7 g

Sat. Fat: 4.4 g

Cholesterol: 19 mg

Protein: 18 g

Sodium: 711 mg

Calcium: 324 mg

Diabetic exchanges: 1 medium-fat meat, 2 starch, 1 vegetable

Spicy Garbanzo Wrap
Yield: 1 serving

1 whole wheat flour tortilla (9-inch round)
1/4 cup plus 2 tablespoons Spicy Garbanzo Spread (see page 260) or ready-made hummus
3 tablespoons coarsely shredded carrots
1/3 cup (packed) fresh spinach leaves

Spoon the garbanzo spread in an even layer over the tortilla, leaving a 1 1/2-inch border on all sides. Layer on the carrots and spinach. Fold the sides in about 1 inch and roll up snugly from the bottom. Cut in half and serve.

Nutritional Facts (per serving):

Calories: 328

Carbohydrates: 52 g

Fiber: 9.7 g

Fat: 8.3 g

Sat. Fat: 1.2 g

Cholesterol: 0 mg

Protein: 13 g

Sodium: 632 mg

Calcium: 176 mg

Diabetic exchanges: 1 lean meat, 2 1/2 starch, 1 vegetable, 1/2 fat

Pressed Spinach Sandwiches
Yield: 2 servings

3 tablespoons thinly sliced scallions or leeks
4 cups (moderately packed) chopped fresh spinach
2 tablespoons chopped black olives
1 tablespoon chopped sun-dried tomatoes
1 tablespoon nonfat or low-fat mayonnaise
3/4 teaspoon Dijon or spicy mustard
4 slices Italian-style multigrain bread (1.1 ounces each)
2 ounces thinly sliced reduced-fat mozzarella, white cheddar, or Swiss cheese
Olive oil cooking spray

Coat a medium-large skillet with cooking spray and add the scallions. Cover and cook over medium heat for a few minutes, or until the scallions start to soften. Add the spinach and cook with the cover on for another minute or two or until wilted. Remove from the heat and toss in the olives, sun-dried tomatoes, mayonnaise, and mustard and stir to mix.

Top two of the bread slices with half of the spinach mixture and half of the cheese. Top with the remaining bread slices. Spray both sides of each sandwich with the cooking spray. Place in a sandwich press or tabletop grill (such as a George Foreman grill) and cook for about 4 minutes, or until the bread is toasted and the cheese is melted. Cut the sandwiches in half and serve hot.

Nutritional Facts (per sandwich):
Calories: 273
Carbohydrates: 36 g
Fiber: 6.4 g
Fat: 8.6 g
Sat. Fat: 3.8 g
Cholesterol: 15 mg
Protein: 16 g
Sodium: 710 mg

Calcium: 342 mg

Diabetic exchanges: I medium-fat meat, 2 starch, I vegetable, I/2 fat

Pita & Portabella Panini
Yield: 2 servings

2 cups sliced baby portabella mushrooms
1/4 teaspoon dried sage
1/8 teaspoon sea salt
1/8 teaspoon ground black pepper
2 whole grain pitas (6-inch rounds)
1/3 cup jarred roasted red bell pepper strips, drained
1/2 cup shredded reduced-fat mozzarella cheese
Olive oil cooking spray

Coat a large nonstick skillet with cooking spray. Add the mushrooms, sage, salt, and pepper and place over medium heat. Cover and cook for 5 to 7 minutes, stirring occasionally, until nicely browned and tender. Remove from the heat and set aside.

Cut the pitas in half and fill each half with one-fourth of the mushrooms, roasted peppers, and cheese. Spray both sides of the pitas with cooking spray. Place the sandwiches in a sandwich press or tabletop grill (such as a George Foreman grill) and cook for about 4 minutes or until the pitas are toasted and the cheese is melted. Cut each pocket in half. Let sit for a couple of minutes before eating, as the mushroom filling may be very hot.

Nutritional Facts (per serving)
Calories: 244
Carbohydrates: 37 g
Fiber: 4.3 g
Fat: 5 g
Sat. Fat: 3.1 g
Cholesterol: 15 mg
Protein: 16 g

Sodium: 427 mg

Calcium: 254 mg

Diabetic exchanges: I medium-fat meat, 2 starch, I vegetable

Unfried Falafel
Yield: 5 servings

15-ounce can chickpeas, drained (reserve a few tablespoons of the liquid)
1/2 cup chopped fresh parsley
1/4 cup chopped yellow onion
2 teaspoons ground cumin
1/2 teaspoon ground coriander
1 1/2 teaspoons crushed garlic
1/4 teaspoon ground black pepper
1/4 teaspoon cayenne pepper
Olive oil cooking spray
2 1/2 whole grain pitas (6-inch rounds), cut in half to make 5 pockets
1 1/4 cups shredded lettuce
10 slices plum tomato

SAUCE
3 tablespoons sesame tahini
2 tablespoons lemon juice
1/2 cup plain nonfat or low-fat Greek-style yogurt
3/4 teaspoon crushed garlic
1/4 teaspoon sea salt

To make the sauce, place the tahini and lemon juice in a small bowl and whisk until smooth. Whisk in the yogurt, garlic, and salt and set aside.

Place the chickpeas, parsley, onion, cumin, coriander, garlic, black pepper, and cayenne pepper in a food processor and process until the mixture is pasty enough to shape into patties. You may need to add 1 to 3 tablespoons of the reserved liquid from the chickpeas to obtain the desired consistency. Shape into 10 patties, each about 2 inches in diameter. Spray the tops of the patties lightly with the cooking spray.

Coat a large nonstick skillet or griddle with the cooking spray and preheat over medium heat until a drop of water sizzles when added. Add the patties to the skillet with the sprayed side up. Cook uncovered for about 3 minutes on each side or until nicely browned. Fill each pita half 1/4 cup of the lettuce, 2 tomato slices, 2 falafel patties, and some of the sauce. Serve hot.

Nutritional Facts (per serving):
Calories: 245
Carbohydrates: 39 g
Fiber: 6.6 g
Fat: 6 g
Sat. Fat: 0.8 g
Cholesterol: 0 mg
Protein: 11 g
Sodium: 345 mg
Calcium: 98 mg
Diabetic exchanges: 1 lean meat, 2 starch, 1 vegetable

Chapter 14:
Main Event Salads

It is hard to beat the ease and versatility of a colorful main dish salad. Many tasty and delicious salads can be created in a matter of minutes, using a wide variety of handy ingredients. Salads are a natural for the AGE-Less Way, since plant foods are naturally very low in AGEs. As a bonus, plant foods are chock full of age-defying nutrients and antioxidants that boost the benefits of your AGE-Less Way.

This chapter offers an array of sensational main dish salads. AGEs are kept within reasonable limits by starting out with generous amounts of wholesome vegetables, fruits, whole grains, pasta, and legumes. Light dressings, herbs, and spices infuse delectable flavors. These recipes feature reduced-fat cheeses as well as lean meats, poultry, and seafood prepared the AGE-Less Way using moist-heat cooking methods.

Perfectly Poached Chicken or Fish

The world's finest cuisines feature delectable poached foods. Poaching is one of the easiest cooking methods and the ultimate method for keeping AGE formation to a minimum. Use this basic recipe for poached chicken or fish as a simple main course or use in salads, sandwiches, and other dishes. For extra flavor, add a few teaspoons of your favorite seasoning to the poaching liquid or try the variations presented below. Note that adding acidic ingredients like lemon or wine to the poaching liquid will reduce AGE formation by about 25-30% more than poaching in plain water or broth.

1. *Start with 4 boneless skinless chicken breast halves or fish fillets. If desired, pound chicken to an even half-inch thickness (this will tenderize the meat, speed cooking time, and increase absorption of flavors from the poaching liquid).*
2. *Place the chicken or fish in a nonstick or non-reactive skillet large enough to hold it in a single layer. Add enough water or broth to submerge the chicken or fish (about 2 cups). Cover the pan and cook over medium heat until the liquid begins to simmer.*
3. *Adjust the heat to maintain a low simmer (the surface of the liquid should bubble every few seconds). Cover and cook chicken for about 15 minutes or until the chicken is cooked through. The thickest part should reach at least 165 degrees F. Cook fish for about 10 minutes per inch-thickness of the fish, or until the fish turns opaque and flakes easily with a fork.*

Variations:

Simply Lemon — Add the juice of 2 lemons (about 4 to 6 tablespoons) to the poaching liquid. Add a few peppercorns or some freshly ground black pepper if desired.

Lemon-Herb — Add the juice of 2 lemons; 1 teaspoon chopped garlic; and 1 teaspoon herbs de Provence, fines herbs, or dried thyme (or several sprigs of fresh herbs) to the poaching liquid.

Mediterranean — Add the juice of 2 lemons, 1 teaspoon chopped garlic, 1 teaspoon dried oregano (or several sprigs of fresh oregano), and 1 tablespoon capers to the poaching liquid.

White Wine — Substitute white wine for half of the poaching water or broth. Add 1 teaspoon of your favorite dried herb or a few sprigs of fresh herbs if desired.

Green Tea & Ginger — Add 5 to 6 thin slices of fresh gingerroot plus the contents of 1 green tea bag to the poaching liquid.

Tips for using poached chicken: Poach a large batch of chicken and freeze the leftovers for later use. When you need chicken for a recipe, simply thaw in the refrigerator overnight and use in the recipe.

For an AGE-Less version of grilled chicken salad, sprinkle both sides of a poached chicken breast with seasoning (such as Cajun or Greek). Coat a nonstick skillet with cooking spray and add the chicken. Cover and cook over medium heat for about 2 minutes per side to heat through. Another option is to place a chicken breast in a nonstick skillet with 1 1/2 tablespoons low-fat vinaigrette salad dressing (such as light balsamic or Italian). Cook and cover for 2 minutes, then cook uncovered for about 1 minute per side, until most of the liquid evaporates and the chicken is heated through and glazed with the dressing.

Lemon-Herb Chicken Salad
Yield: 4 servings

2 cups diced Lemon-Herb poached chicken (see page 170)
1/3 cup finely chopped celery
1/3 cup thinly sliced scallions
1 1/2 tablespoons finely chopped fresh parsley or 1 1/2 teaspoons dried
1/2 to 1 tablespoon finely chopped fresh dill or chives or 1/2 to 1 teaspoon dried
1/3 cup nonfat or light sour cream
1/3 cup nonfat or light mayonnaise

Place the chicken, celery, scallions, and herbs in a medium bowl, and toss to mix. Add the sour cream and mayonnaise and stir to mix well. Serve over a bed of fresh salad greens or use as a sandwich filling.

Nutritional Facts (per 2/3-cup serving):
Calories: 137
Carbohydrates: 7 g
Fiber: 0.4 g
Fat: 2.2 g
Sat. Fat: 0.6 g

Cholesterol: 54 mg
Protein: 21 g
Sodium: 220 mg
Calcium: 48 mg
Diabetic exchanges: 2 1/2 lean meat, 1/2 carbohydrate

Artichoke Chicken Salad
Yield: 4 servings

2 cups diced Lemon-Herb or Mediterranean Poached Chicken (see page 170)
1 1/2 cups marinated artichoke hearts, drained and chopped
3/4 cup chopped red onion
1/4 cup plus 2 tablespoons nonfat or light mayonnaise

Combine the chicken, artichoke hearts, and onion in a bowl. Add the mayonnaise and toss to mix. Add a little more mayonnaise if needed. Serve immediately. If desired, serve over a bed of Boston lettuce leaves, in a tomato cup, or in a whole grain pita or wrap.

Nutritional Facts (per 1-cup serving):
Calories: 170
Carbohydrates: 13 g
Fiber: 2.4 g
Fat: 2.9 g
Sat. Fat: 0.7 g
Cholesterol: 55 mg
Protein: 23 g
Sodium: 425 mg
Calcium: 15 mg
Diabetic exchanges: 2 1/2 lean meat, 1 carbohydrate

Fruited Chicken & Rice Salad
Yield: 6 servings

3 cups cooked brown rice, chilled*
2 cups diced Green Tea and Ginger poached chicken (see page 170)

1/2 cup canned water chestnuts, drained and chopped
1/2 cup thinly sliced celery
1/3 cup thinly sliced scallions
1/2 cup canned mandarin oranges, drained
1/2 cup pineapple tidbits canned in juice, drained
1/3 cup slivered almonds

DRESSING
1/2 cup plus 2 tablespoons light lemon yogurt
1/2 cup plus 2 tablespoons nonfat or light mayonnaise
1/2 teaspoon curry powder (optional)

Combine the rice, chicken, water chestnuts, celery, scallions, oranges, pineapple, and almonds in a large bowl and toss to mix. Combine the dressing ingredients and stir to mix. Add the dressing to the rice mixture and toss to mix. Serve immediately or cover and chill until ready to serve. Serve on a bed of mixed salad greens if desired.

Nutritional Facts (per 1 1/3-cup serving):
Calories: 281
Carbohydrates: 39 g
Fiber: 3.7 g
Fat: 5.1 g
Sat. Fat: 0.8 g
Cholesterol: 40 mg
Protein: 20 g
Sodium: 246 mg
Calcium: 90 mg
Diabetic exchanges: 2 lean meat, 2 starch, 1/2 fruit

*Prepare 1 cup uncooked brown rice according to package directions.

Couscous Chicken Salad
Yield: 5 servings

3 cups prepared whole wheat couscous, chilled*
2 cups diced Simply Lemon or White Wine poached chicken (see page 170)
3/4 cup thinly sliced celery
3/4 cup frozen green peas
1/3 cup thinly sliced scallions

DRESSING
1/2 cup nonfat or light mayonnaise
1/3 cup nonfat or light sour cream
1/4 cup orange juice
1 teaspoon Dijon mustard
1 tablespoon finely chopped fresh dill or 1 teaspoon dried
1/4 teaspoon ground black pepper

Combine the couscous, chicken, celery, peas, and scallions in a large bowl and toss to mix. Combine the dressing ingredients in a small bowl and stir to mix. Add the dressing to the couscous mixture and toss to mix. Cover and chill for at least 1 hour before serving. Serve on a bed of mixed salad greens if desired.

Nutritional Facts (per 1 1/4-cup serving):
Calories: 275
Carbohydrates: 37 g
Fiber: 6 g
Fat: 3.5 g
Sat. Fat: 0.7 g
Cholesterol: 50 mg
Protein: 24 g
Sodium: 321 mg
Calcium: 66 mg
Diabetic exchanges: 2 lean meat, 2 carbohydrate

*Prepare 1 cup dry couscous according to package directions.

Chicken Salad with Grapes & Walnuts
Yield: 4 servings

2 cups diced Simply Lemon or White Wine poached chicken (see page 170)
1 cup seedless red grapes
1/3 cup thinly sliced celery
1/3 cup sliced scallions
1/3 cup chopped walnuts or pecans

DRESSING
1/3 cup nonfat or light sour cream or Greek style yogurt
1/3 cup nonfat or light mayonnaise
1 to 1 1/2 teaspoons curry powder (optional)

Combine the chicken, grapes, celery, scallions, and nuts in a medium bowl. Combine the dressing ingredients in a small bowl, and stir to mix. Add the dressing to the chicken mixture and toss to mix. Serve on a bed of fresh salad greens or in a whole grain pita pocket or wrap if desired.

Nutritional Facts (per 1-cup serving):
Calories: 229
Carbohydrates: 15 g
Fiber: 1.3 g
Fat: 8.2 g
Sat. Fat: 1 g
Cholesterol: 55 mg
Protein: 24 g
Sodium: 220 mg
Calcium: 56 mg
Diabetic exchanges: 2 1/2 lean meat, 1 carbohydrate, 1 fat

Mediterranean Chopped Salad
Yield: 2 servings

6 cups chopped romaine lettuce
1 cup chopped tomato
1 cup chopped cucumber
1/2 cup chopped red onion
1 cup diced Mediterranean poached chicken (see page 170), or substitute poached or canned salmon or tuna
1/3 cup chopped Kalamata or black olives
1 1/2 teaspoons capers, finely minced
1/4 cup crumbled reduced-fat feta cheese
1 1/2 tablespoons extra virgin olive oil
1 1/2 tablespoons red wine vinegar
Freshly ground black pepper

Combine the lettuce, tomato, cucumber, onion, chicken, olives, capers, and feta cheese in a large bowl. Drizzle the oil and vinegar over the salad and sprinkle with some pepper. Toss to mix. Serve immediately.

Nutritional Facts (per serving):
Calories: 316
Carbohydrates: 16 g
Fiber: 5.8 g
Fat: 17 g
Sat. Fat: 3.6 g
Cholesterol: 58 mg
Protein: 28 g
Sodium: 521 mg
Calcium: 153 mg
Diabetic exchanges: 3 lean meat, 3 vegetable, 2 fat

Chipotle Chicken Salad
Yield: 4 servings

10 cups shredded romaine lettuce
2 cups diced or shredded poached chicken
1 cup chopped tomatoes
1 cup diced avocado
1/2 cup chopped red onion
1 cup canned black beans, rinsed and drained
1 cup frozen corn, thawed

DRESSING
1/2 cup nonfat or light sour cream
1/4 cup chunky-style salsa
1 tablespoon finely chopped canned chipotle chili in adobo sauce
1/2 teaspoon ground cumin
Scant 1/4 teaspoon sea salt

Place the lettuce, chicken, tomatoes, avocado, onion, beans, and corn in a large bowl. Combine the dressing ingredients and stir to mix. Add the dressing to the salad and toss to mix. Serve immediately.

Nutritional Facts (per serving):
Calories: 318
Carbohydrates: 32 g
Fiber: 10 g
Fat: 8.9 g
Sat. Fat: 1.7 g
Cholesterol: 54 mg
Protein: 30 g
Sodium: 583 mg
Calcium: 123 mg
Diabetic exchanges: 3 lean meat, 3 vegetable, 1 starch, 1 fat

Chicken & Broccoli Pasta Salad
Yield: 4 servings

6 ounces whole grain penne or rotini pasta
2 1/2 cups small fresh broccoli florets (about 1/2-inch pieces)
2 cups diced poached chicken
2/3 cup sliced scallions
1/2 cup coarsely shredded carrots
1/4 cup chopped walnuts (optional)
Freshly ground black pepper

DRESSING
2/3 cup nonfat or light mayonnaise
1/3 cup nonfat or light sour cream
1 tablespoon finely chopped fresh dill or 2 teaspoons dried

Cook the pasta according to package directions until almost al dente. Add the broccoli to the pot and cook for 1 minute more, or until the broccoli is crisp-tender and the pasta is done. Drain the pasta and broccoli, rinse with cool water, and drain again.

Place the pasta mixture in a large bowl, and add the chicken, scallions, carrots, and walnuts (if using). Sprinkle with some pepper and toss to mix. Combine the mayonnaise, sour cream, and dill in a small bowl and stir to mix. Add to the salad, and toss to mix. Cover and chill for at least 1 hour before serving.

Nutritional Facts (per 2-cup serving):
Calories: 301
Carbohydrates: 43 g
Fiber: 5.1 g
Fat: 2.9 g
Sat. Fat: 0.7 g
Cholesterol: 54 mg
Protein: 28 g
Sodium: 370 mg

Calcium: 89 mg

Diabetic exchanges: 2 1/2 lean meat, 2 starch, 1 1/2 vegetable

Layered Seafood Salad
Yield: 5 servings

4 ounces whole grain penne or rotini pasta
6 cups shredded romaine lettuce
3 hard-boiled eggs, coarsely chopped
2 cups boiled or steamed shrimp, lump crabmeat, or canned water-packed
tuna or salmon
1 1/4 cups frozen green peas, thawed
1 cup nonfat or light mayonnaise
1/4 cup nonfat or light sour cream
3/4 cup shredded reduced-fat cheddar cheese
1/2 cup diced seeded plum tomato
1/4 cup sliced scallions
2 tablespoons finely chopped fresh dill or 2 teaspoons dried dill

Cook the pasta according to package directions. Drain, rinse with cold water, and drain again. Spread the pasta over the bottom of a 3-quart glass bowl. Layer on the lettuce, peas, eggs, and your choice of shrimp, crab, tuna, or salmon. Combine the mayonnaise and sour cream and stir to mix. Spread over the layer of peas.

Cover the bowl and refrigerate for several hours or overnight. Just before serving, top the salad with the cheese, tomatoes, scallions, and dill. Toss the salad and serve immediately.

Nutritional Facts (per serving):
Calories: 301
Carbohydrates: 36 g
Fiber: 5.3 g
Fat: 7 g
Sat. Fat: 3 g
Cholesterol: 247 mg

Protein: 27 g
Sodium: 687 mg
Calcium: 233 mg
Diabetic exchanges: 3 lean meat, 1 1/2 starch, 1 1/2 vegetable

Shrimp Cobb Salad
Yield: 2 servings

6 cups chopped romaine lettuce
16 medium peeled boiled or steamed shrimp (about 5 ounces)
3/4 cup chopped tomatoes
3/4 cup chopped cucumber
1/2 cup chopped red onion
2 hard-boiled eggs, sliced
Freshly ground black pepper

DRESSING
1/4 cup light blue cheese crumbles
2 tablespoons nonfat or light sour cream
1/2 teaspoon crushed garlic
1 1/2 tablespoons white wine
1/4 cup nonfat or light mayonnaise

To make the dressing, combine the blue cheese, sour cream, and gar-lic in a small bowl and stir to mix. Use a fork to finely mash about half of the blue cheese. Stir in the wine and then the mayonnaise. Add a little more wine if the dressing seems too thick. Set aside.

Divide the lettuce between 2 large salad bowls or plates. Arrange half of the shrimp, tomatoes, cucumber, onion, and egg over the top of each salad. Sprinkle with pepper and serve immediately accompanied by the dressing.

Nutritional Facts (per serving):
Calories: 281
Carbohydrates: 20 g

Fiber: 4.6 g

Fat: 9.8 g

Sat. Fat: 4.2 g

Cholesterol: 362 mg

Protein: 28 g

Sodium: 621 mg

Calcium: 209 mg

Diabetic exchanges: 2 1/2 lean meat, 1 medium-fat meat, 3 vegetable

Dilled Salmon Salad
Yield: 4 servings

1 cup uncooked whole wheat orzo (about 6 ounces)
1 1/4 cups poached, steamed, or canned (drained) salmon
3/4 cup chopped peeled seeded cucumber
1/2 cup seeded chopped plum tomato
1/2 cup thinly sliced scallions
1 to 1 1/2 tablespoons finely chopped fresh dill or 1 to 1 1/2 teaspoons dried dill
Freshly ground black pepper

DRESSING
2 tablespoons extra virgin olive oil
1 tablespoon plus 1 teaspoon lemon juice
2 teaspoons Dijon mustard
1/4 teaspoon sea salt

Cook the orzo according to package directions. Drain, rinse with cool water, and drain again. Place the orzo in a large bowl. Add the salmon, cucumber, tomato, scallions, and dill. Sprinkle with some pepper. Set aside.

Combine the dressing ingredients in a small bowl and stir to mix. Pour over the salad and toss gently to mix. Serve immediately or cover and chill until ready to serve. Serve over a bed of mixed baby salad greens or Boston lettuce if desired.

Nutritional Facts (per 1 1/3-cup serving):

Calories: 289

Carbohydrates: 32 g

Fiber: 4.4 g

Fat: 11 g

Sat. Fat: 1.8 g

Cholesterol: 25 mg

Protein: 19 g

Sodium: 240 mg

Potassium: 388 mg

Calcium: 58 mg

Diabetic exchanges: 1 1/2 lean meat, 2 carbohydrate, 1 fat

Orzo-Crab Salad
Yield: 5 servings

1 cup uncooked whole wheat orzo (about 6 ounces)
2 cups steamed or boiled crabmeat
1 cup chopped canned (drained) artichoke hearts
3/4 cup chopped seeded plum tomato
1/2 cup thinly sliced scallions

DRESSING
1/4 cup nonfat or light mayonnaise
1/4 cup light Italian or olive oil vinaigrette salad dressing

Cook the orzo according to package directions. Drain, rinse with cool water, and drain again. Combine the orzo, crab, artichokes, tomato, and scallions in a large bowl. Add the mayonnaise and salad dressing, and toss to mix. Cover and refrigerate for at least 1 hour before serving. Serve on a bed of mixed salad greens if desired.

Nutritional Facts (per 1 1/3-cup serving):

Calories: 252

Carbohydrates: 32 g

Fiber: 5.9 g
Cholesterol: 30 mg
Fat: 6.4 g
Sat. fat: 0.3 g
Protein: 16.6 g
Sodium: 692 mg
Calcium: 64 mg
Diabetic exchanges: 2 lean meat, 1 1/2 starch, 1 vegetable

Summertime Crab Salad
Yield: 4 servings

2 cups steamed or boiled crabmeat (about 10 ounces)
1 1/2 cups frozen whole kernel corn, thawed
1/2 cup sliced scallions
1 cup grape tomatoes, halved or quartered
1/4 cup finely chopped fresh basil

DRESSING
2 tablespoons white wine vinegar
2 tablespoons lemon juice
2 tablespoons extra virgin olive oil
1 teaspoon frozen orange juice concentrate
Scant 1/2 teaspoon sea salt
1/4 teaspoon ground black pepper

Place the crabmeat, corn, scallions, tomatoes, and basil in a large bowl. Set aside. Combine the dressing ingredients and whisk until smooth. Pour the dressing over the salad and toss to mix. Serve immediately or cover and chill. Serve over a bed of fresh spinach leaves or mixed baby salad greens if desired.

Nutritional Facts (per 1 1/4-cup serving):
Calories: 194
Carbohydrates: 17 g

Fiber: 2.4 g
Fat: 8.7 g
Sat. Fat: 1.2 g
Cholesterol: 59 mg
Protein: 14.5 g
Sodium: 403 mg
Calcium: 80 mg
Diabetic exchanges: 2 1/2 lean meat, 1 starch

Tabbouleh Tuna Salad
Yield: 5 servings

3 cups bulgur wheat, chilled*
1 cup chopped fresh tomatoes
1 cup chopped peeled and seeded cucumber
1/2 cup sliced scallions
1/2 cup finely chopped fresh parsley
2 cans (6 ounces each) chunk tuna in water, drained

DRESSING
3 tablespoons lemon juice
3 tablespoons extra virgin olive oil
1/4 teaspoon sea salt
1/4 teaspoon ground black pepper

Place the bulgur wheat, tomatoes, cucumber, scallions, and parsley in a large bowl. Combine the dressing ingredients in a small bowl and whisk to mix. Pour the dressing over the salad and toss to mix. Add the tuna and toss gently. Cover and chill for 1 to 3 hours before serving. If desired, serve on a bed of fresh salad greens and top each serving with a sprinkling of reduced-fat feta cheese.

Nutritional Facts (per 1 1/3-cup serving):
Calories: 256
Carbohydrates: 24 g

Fiber: 6 g
Fat: 9.1 g
Sat. Fat: 1.3 g
Cholesterol: 20 mg
Protein: 21 g
Sodium: 353 mg
Calcium: 39 mg
Diabetic exchanges: 2 lean meat, 1 1/2 starch, 1 vegetable, 1 fat

*Prepare 1 cup dry bulgur wheat according to package directions.

Salmon Salad Nicoise
Yield: 4 servings

3/4 pound red-skinned new potatoes, cut into 3/4-inch chunks (about 2 1/2 cups)
1/2 cup plus 2 tablespoons light olive oil vinaigrette salad dressing
2 cups fresh green beans (1 to 1 1/2-inch pieces)
8 cups torn Boston or romaine lettuce
1 cup cherry tomatoes, halved
4 slices red onion, cut into quarter-rings
2 cans (6 ounces each) water-packed boneless, skinless salmon or 1 1/2 cups poached or steamed salmon (or substitute canned tuna)
2 hard-boiled eggs, quartered lengthwise
1/3 cup Kalamata olives, pitted and coarsely chopped
2 tablespoons capers

Steam the potatoes for about 10 minutes or until tender. Place in a bowl, and toss with 2 tablespoons of the dressing. Set aside. Steam the green beans for about 4 minutes or until crisp-tender. Place in a bowl of ice water, let sit for about 30 seconds, and then drain very well. Toss the green beans with 2 tablespoons of the dressing and set aside.

Place the lettuce, tomatoes, and onion in a large bowl. Pour on the remaining dressing and toss to mix. Place one-fourth of the salad mix on a dinner plate and mound one-fourth of the salmon in the center. Mound one-fourth of the potatoes and green beans on opposite sides of the salmon. Place 2 egg quarters on opposite sides of the salmon. Repeat to make 3 more salads. Sprinkle each salad with one-fourth of the olives and capers and serve immediately.

Nutritional Facts (per serving):
Calories: 332
Carbohydrates: 30 g
Fiber: 7 g
Fat: 16 g
Sat. Fat: 2.7 g
Cholesterol: 139 mg
Protein: 20 g
Sodium: 600 mg
Calcium: 188 mg
Diabetic exchanges: 3 lean meat, 1 starch, 3 vegetable, 1 fat

Couscous Shrimp Salad
Yield: 5 servings

3 cups prepared whole wheat couscous, chilled*
2 cups peeled boiled or steamed medium-size shrimp
3 cups (moderately packed) thinly sliced fresh spinach leaves
3/4 cup thinly sliced scallions
1/2 cup finely chopped fresh parsley
1 cup halved grape tomatoes
1/4 cup crumbled reduced-fat feta cheese

DRESSING
1/4 cup lemon juice
3 tablespoons extra virgin olive oil
1 1/2 teaspoons crushed garlic
1/2 teaspoon sea salt
1/2 teaspoon ground black pepper

Place the couscous, shrimp, spinach, scallions, parsley, tomatoes, and feta cheese in a large bowl. Combine the dressing ingredients in a bowl and whisk to mix. Pour the dressing over the salad and toss to mix. Serve immediately or cover and refrigerate until ready to serve.

Nutritional Facts (per 1 1/3-cup serving):
Calories: 331
Carbohydrates: 41 g
Fiber: 7.2 g
Fat: 10.5 g
Sat. Fat: 1.8 g
Cholesterol: 112 mg
Protein: 21 g
Sodium: 459 mg
Calcium: 97 mg
Diabetic exchanges: 2 1/2 lean meat, 2 starch, 1 vegetable, 1 fat

*Prepare 1 cup dry couscous according to package directions.

Tuna Salad with Pasta & Roasted Red Peppers
Yield: 3 servings

6 ounces whole grain penne or rotini pasta
6-ounce can tuna in water, drained
1/2 cup thinly sliced scallions
1/4 cup chopped black olives
3/4 cup jarred roasted red bell peppers, drained and diced
1/4 cup nonfat or light mayonnaise
1 teaspoon crushed garlic
1 teaspoon dried basil or 1 tablespoon fresh
1/4 teaspoon ground black pepper

Cook the pasta according to package directions. Drain, rinse with cool water, and drain again. Place the pasta, tuna, scallions, olives, and 1/2 cup of the red bell peppers in a large bowl.

Combine the remaining red bell peppers, mayonnaise, garlic, basil, and black pepper in a mini food processor or mini blender jar and process until smooth. Add to the pasta mixture and toss to mix. Cover and chill for at least 1 hour before serving. Toss in a little more mayonnaise just before serving if needed. Serve over a bed of romaine lettuce if desired.

Nutritional Facts (per 1 2/3-cup serving):
Calories: 291
Carbohydrates: 45 g
Fiber: 5.3 g
Fat: 3.7 g
Sat. Fat: 0.8 g
Cholesterol: 24 mg
Protein: 21 g
Sodium: 460 mg
Calcium: 53 mg
Diabetic exchanges: 2 lean meat, 2 1/2 starch, 1 vegetable

Cannellini Tuna Salad
Yield: 3 servings

6-ounce can tuna in water, drained
15-ounce can cannellini or white beans, rinsed and well drained
1 cup marinated artichoke hearts, drained and coarsely chopped (reserve the marinade)
1/3 cup chopped red onion
1/4 cup chopped fresh parsley
Freshly ground black pepper

Combine the tuna, beans, artichoke hearts, onion, and parsley in a large bowl. Add 1/4 cup of the reserved marinade and sprinkle with pepper to taste; toss gently to mix. Serve immediately or cover and chill. Toss in a little more marinade just before serving if needed.

Nutritional Facts (per 1 1/8-cup serving):
Calories: 255
Carbohydrates: 27 g
Fiber: 7.7 g
Fat: 7.3 g
Sat. Fat: 0.7 g
Cholesterol: 24 mg
Protein: 21 g
Sodium: 608 mg
Calcium: 58 mg
Diabetic exchanges: 3 lean meat, 1 1/2 starch

Sesame Noodle Salad
Yield: 5 servings

2 cups diced extra-firm tofu, or substitute steamed or boiled shrimp or poached chicken
6 ounces whole grain spaghetti or Japanese soba noodles, broken into 3-inch lengths
1 1/4 cups fresh broccoli florets (1/2-inch pieces)
1/2 cup grated carrot
1/2 cup sliced scallions
1/2 cup cooked shelled edamame or frozen (thawed) green peas
3 tablespoons non-toasted sesame seeds

DRESSING
3 tablespoons rice vinegar
3 tablespoons reduced-sodium soy sauce
3 tablespoons orange juice
2 tablespoons canola oil
1 tablespoon honey
1 tablespoon finely grated fresh ginger
1/2 teaspoon ground white pepper

Combine all of the dressing ingredients in a medium bowl and whisk to mix well. Add the tofu and toss gently to coat with the dressing. Set aside.

Cook the noodles according to package directions. Drain, rinse with cool water and drain again. Place the noodles in a large bowl. Add the broccoli, carrots, scallions, edamame or peas, and sesame seeds. Pour the dressing and tofu over the salad. Toss gently to mix. Cover and chill for at least one hour before serving.

Nutritional Facts (per 1 1/2-cup serving):
Calories: 332
Carbohydrates: 33 g
Fiber: 8.5 g
Fat: 13.6 g
Sat. Fat: 1.9 g
Cholesterol: 0 mg
Protein: 26 g
Sodium: 395 mg
Calcium: 754 mg
Diabetic exchanges: 2 medium-fat meat, 1 1/2 starch, 1 vegetable, 1 fat

Great Garbanzo Salad
Yield: 4 servings

1/2 cup uncooked whole wheat orzo
1 cup canned chickpeas (garbanzo beans), drained
3/4 cup diced seedless cucumber
3/4 cup chopped plum tomato
1/2 cup chopped red onion
1/4 cup plus 2 tablespoons finely chopped fresh basil
1 cup diced fresh mozzarella cheese

DRESSING
2 tablespoons extra virgin olive oil
2 tablespoons white wine vinegar

1/4 teaspoon sea salt
1/4 teaspoon ground black pepper

Cook the orzo according to package directions. Drain, rinse with cool water, and drain well. Place the orzo in a large bowl and add the chickpeas, cucumber, tomato, onion, and basil.

Combine the dressing ingredients and whisk to mix. Pour the dressing over the salad and toss to mix. Toss in the mozzarella cheese. Chill for at least 1 hour before serving. Serve over a bed of fresh spinach or romaine if desired.

Nutritional Facts (per 1 1/8-cup serving):
Calories: 304
Carbohydrates: 33 g
Fiber: 7.1 g
Fat: 14 g
Sat. Fat: 5 g
Cholesterol: 22 mg
Protein: 11.4 g
Sodium: 369 mg
Calcium: 212 mg
Diabetic exchanges: 1 1/2 lean meat, 1 1/2 starch, 1 vegetable, 1 1/2 fat

Colorful Lentil Salad
Yield: 5 servings

3 cups cooked brown lentils*
1 cup (packed) chopped fresh parsley
1 cup sliced scallions
1 cup grated carrots

DRESSING
3 tablespoons extra virgin olive oil
2 tablespoons lemon juice
1 1/2 teaspoons crushed garlic

3/4 teaspoon Dijon mustard
3/4 teaspoon sea salt
1/2 teaspoon ground black pepper

Place the lentils, parsley, scallions, and carrots in a large bowl. Combine the dressing ingredients and whisk to mix. Pour the dressing over the salad and toss to mix. Cover and chill for at least 1 hour before serving.

Nutritional Facts (per 1-cup serving):
Calories: 237
Carbohydrates: 29 g
Fiber: 11 g
Fat: 9 g
Sat. Fat: 1.3 g
Cholesterol: 0 mg
Protein: 11.8 g
Sodium: 384 mg
Calcium: 63 mg
Diabetic exchanges: 1 lean meat, 1 starch, 1 vegetable, 2 fat

*Place 1 cup dried lentils and 3 cups water in a 2-quart pot and bring to a boil. Reduce the heat to maintain a simmer. Cover and cook for 25 to 30 minutes or until tender but not mushy. Drain off any excess liquid. Cool before adding to the salad.

Chapter 15: Easy Main Courses

The main course, or entrée, typically adds more AGEs to our daily diet than any other food. This is because the main course often features a large portion of meat or poultry cooked with high dry heat methods such as grilling, broiling, frying, or roasting. But even meatless main courses can be loaded with AGEs if made with gobs of high-fat cheese, butter, and oil.

Fortunately, AGE-Less entrees can be tasty, filling, and a snap to prepare. In fact, the two magic meal words in the average working household—fast and easy—are also pivotal to the AGE-Less Way. Short cooking times and moist cooking methods (such as poaching, steaming, and stewing), which require very little attention, are the keys to making AGE-Less meals. Convenient oven-braised and slow cooker meals can also fit the bill. Moreover, many family favorites such as meatloaf, meatballs, skillet dinners, and even tacos can be enjoyed on the AGE-Less Way.

These AGE-Less main courses feature right-size portions of lean protein along with nutrient-rich vegetables and wholesome whole grains. Creative use of acidic ingredients such as lemon juice, wine, and tomatoes along with flavorful herbs enhance the flavor of foods instead of age-accelerating AGEs.

As you peruse this chapter, keep in mind that you will find many more delicious main courses in other chapters this book. A selection of savory soups and stews, hearty sandwiches, and main dish salads can be found in Chapter 12, 13, and 14.

Asian-Style Steamed Chicken with Cilantro Sauce
Yield: 4 servings

1 green tea bag
4 medium-large collard green, kale, or Chinese cabbage leaves
4 boneless skinless chicken breasts (4 ounces each), pounded to an even
1/2-inch thickness
2 tablespoons matchstick-size pieces fresh peeled gingerroot

SAUCE
1 tablespoon canola or non-toasted sesame oil
2 teaspoons crushed garlic
2 tablespoons reduced-sodium soy sauce
2 teaspoons rice vinegar
1 teaspoon Asian-style chili sauce with garlic
1/2 cup finely chopped fresh cilantro

Cut open the tea bag and pour the contents into a 6-quart pot. Add a steamer basket and pour in enough water to reach within 1/2 inch of the bottom of the basket. Line the basket with the collard, kale, or cabbage leaves. Top each leaf with a chicken breast and cover each piece of chicken with one-fourth of the ginger.

Cover the pot and bring to a boil. Steam for about 15 minutes or until the thickest part of the chicken reaches an internal temperature of at least 165 degrees F. Remove 1/4 cup of the liquid from the pot (excluding the tea leaves) and set aside to use in the sauce. Set the chicken aside to keep warm.

To make the sauce, place the oil and garlic in a small skillet. Cook over medium heat for about 30 seconds or just until the garlic begins to turn color and smells fragrant. Add the 1/4 cup liquid from the pot along with the soy sauce, vinegar, chili sauce, and cilantro. Let the sauce come to a boil and cook for about a minute to reduce in volume by about one-third. Serve the chicken on the collard, kale, or cabbage leaves and drizzle with sauce.

Nutritional Facts (per serving):

Calories: 169

Carbohydrates: 2 g

Fiber: 1 g

Fat: 4.9 g

Sat. Fat: 0.6 g

Cholesterol: 66 mg

Protein: 27 g

Sodium: 383 mg

Calcium: 39 mg

Diabetic exchanges: 3 lean meat, 1 fat

Chicken Dijon
Yield: 4 servings

4 sheets of aluminum foil (12-inch squares) or parchment paper (15-inch squares)
2 cups sliced fresh mushrooms
1 medium yellow onion, thinly sliced and separated into rings
1/4 cup dry white wine
Scant 1/4 teaspoon sea salt
Freshly ground black pepper
4 boneless skinless chicken breasts (4 ounces each), pounded to an even 1/2-inch thickness
3 tablespoons Dijon mustard
1 tablespoon finely chopped fresh rosemary or 1 teaspoon dried

Preheat the oven to 350 degrees F. Lay the squares of foil or parchment on a flat surface and center one-fourth of the mushrooms and onions on the lower half of each square. Drizzle the vegetables on each square with 1 tablespoon of wine and sprinkle with some of the salt and pepper. Top the vegetable mixture on each square with a piece of chicken. Spread one-fourth of the mustard over each piece of chicken and sprinkle with the rosemary. Fold the top part of the foil or parchment over the lower part. Double-fold the edges together to tightly seal the packets.

Lay the packets on a large baking sheet and bake for 30 minutes, until cooked through. Let the packets sit for 5 minutes before opening. Open with care, as steam will escape. Serve the chicken, vegetables, and juices over brown rice or whole wheat couscous if desired.

Nutritional Facts (per serving):
Calories: 159
Carbohydrates: 5 g
Fiber: 1.1 g
Fat: 2.6 g
Sat. Fat: 0.5 g
Cholesterol: 66 mg
Protein: 28 g
Sodium: 505 mg
Calcium: 38 mg
Diabetic exchanges: 3 lean meat, 1 vegetable

Chicken & Vegetables en Papillote
Yield: 4 servings

1 medium-large zucchini
1 large carrot
1/2 cup thin slices leek or 8 slices yellow onion, separated into rings
1/4 teaspoon sea salt
Ground black pepper
1 teaspoon fines herbes or herbes de Provence
4 pieces of aluminum foil (12-inch squares) or parchment paper (15-inch squares)
4 boneless skinless chicken breasts (4 ounces each), pounded to an even 1/2-inch thickness
1 1/2 tablespoons Dijon mustard
1 1/2 tablespoons dry white wine

Preheat the oven to 350 degrees F. Using a potato peeler, cut the zucchini and carrot into thin, wide ribbons. Place the ribbons in a bowl and add the leeks or onion, salt, pepper, and half of the herbs. Toss to mix. Lay the squares of foil or parchment on a flat surface and center one-fourth of the vegetable mixture on the lower part of each square.

Top the vegetable mixture on each square with a piece of chicken. Combine the mustard, wine, and remaining herbs and stir to mix. Spread one-fourth of the mustard mixture over each piece of chicken. Fold the top part of the foil or parchment over the lower part and double-fold the edges together to tightly seal the packets.

Lay the packets on a large baking sheet and bake for 25 minutes, until the chicken is cooked through. Let the packets sit for 5 minutes before opening. Open with care, as steam will escape. Serve the chicken, vegetables, and juices over brown rice or whole wheat couscous if desired.

Nutritional Facts (per serving):
Calories: 156
Carbohydrates: 6 g
Fiber: 1.3 g
Fat: 2 g
Sat. Fat: 0.4 g
Cholesterol: 66 mg
Protein: 28 g
Sodium: 374 mg
Calcium: 41 mg
Diabetic exchanges: 3 lean meat, 1 vegetable

Chicken & Barley Risotto
Yield: 5 servings:

3/4 pound boneless skinless chicken breast, cut into 1-inch pieces
3 cups sliced fresh mushrooms
1 medium yellow onion, cut into thin wedges
1 cup pearl barley

2 1/2 cups chicken broth
1/2 cup dry white wine
1/2 cup V-8 vegetable juice
2 teaspoons crushed garlic
1 teaspoon dried marjoram or thyme
Scant 1/2 teaspoon ground black pepper
3/4 cup frozen green peas

Coat a large, deep nonstick skillet or 4-quart pot with cooking spray and preheat over medium heat. Add the chicken and cook for a couple of minutes, or just enough to seal the meat and lightly brown in a few spots. Add the remaining ingredients except for the peas.

Bring to a boil then reduce the heat to maintain a simmer. Cover and cook for about 45 minutes, stirring occasionally, until the barley is tender and most of the liquid is absorbed. Add a little more broth if needed. Add the peas and cook with the cover on for 5 more minutes. Serve hot.

Nutritional Facts (per 1 1/3-cup serving):
Calories: 279
Carbohydrates: 40 g
Fiber: 8.5 g
Fat: 1.6 g
Sat. Fat: 0.4 g
Cholesterol: 39 mg
Protein: 23 g
Sodium: 576 mg
Calcium: 44 mg
Diabetic exchanges: 2 lean meat, 2 starch, 1 vegetable

Moroccan Meatballs with Sweet Onion Sauce
Yield: 4 servings

1 pound 96% lean ground chicken, turkey, or lamb
1/4 cup uncooked whole wheat couscous

1/4 teaspoon sea salt
1/4 teaspoon ground black pepper
3/4 cup finely chopped fresh parsley
1 1/2 teaspoons Moroccan spice blend*
3 cups thin wedges yellow onion
1 1/4 cups chicken broth
10-ounce can Rotelle tomatoes with green chilies
2 teaspoons unbleached flour
1/4 cup plus 1 tablespoon golden raisins

Place the ground meat, couscous, salt, and pepper in a large bowl. Add 1/2 cup of the parsley and 1 teaspoon of the Moroccan spice blend and mix well. Shape into 20 meatballs, each about 1 1/2 inches in diameter. Set aside.

Coat a large deep skillet with cooking spray. Add the onions, 1/4 cup of the broth, and remaining 1/2 teaspoon of Moroccan seasoning and place over medium heat. Cover and cook for about 8 minutes, shaking the pan occasionally, until the onions soften. Add a little water, if needed, to prevent scorching.

Combine the non-drained tomatoes, remaining 1 cup of broth, and the flour in a blender and blend until smooth. Add to the skillet and stir to mix. Cover and bring to a boil over medium heat, stirring occasionally. Add the meatballs to the skillet and adjust the heat to maintain a simmer. Cover and cook for 20 minutes, turning the meatballs after 5 minutes. Stir in the raisins and simmer for 10 minutes more. Serve hot, topping each serving with some of the remaining parsley.

Nutritional Facts (per serving):
Calories: 294
Carbohydrate: 36 g
Fiber: 5.4 g
Fat: 5.7 g
Sat. Fat: 1.1 g
Cholesterol: 90 mg

Protein: 27 g
Sodium: 647 mg
Calcium: 82 mg
Diabetic exchanges: 3 lean meat, 2 carbohydrate

*Purchase a ready-made spice blend or mix together: 2 teaspoons each ground cumin and ginger; 1 teaspoon each ground coriander, turmeric, cinnamon, allspice, and black pepper; and 1/2 teaspoon each ground cloves and cayenne pepper. Store leftover spice in an airtight container.

Saffron Chicken & Orzo
Yield: 5 servings

4 boneless skinless chicken breasts (4 ounces each)
2 cups chicken broth
1 cup dry white wine
2 teaspoons crushed garlic
3/4 teaspoon dried oregano
1/2 teaspoon ground black pepper
1 tablespoon olive oil
3/4 cup chopped yellow onion
1 1/2 cups uncooked whole grain orzo (about 9 ounces)
3/4 cup chopped plum tomato
Scant 1/2 teaspoon loosely packed saffron threads
3/4 cup frozen green peas

Place the chicken in a large deep nonstick skillet and add the broth, wine, garlic, oregano, and pepper. Cover and bring to a boil. Reduce the heat to maintain a simmer and cook for 20 minutes. Remove the chicken and set aside. Measure the liquid in the skillet and pour into a large bowl. If necessary, add enough water to bring the volume to 3 cups. Set aside.

Add the olive oil and onion to the skillet. Cover and place over medium heat. Cook for several minutes, shaking the skillet occasionally, until the onion starts to soften. Add the orzo, tomato, reserved poaching liquid, and saffron and bring to a boil. Reduce the heat to medium-low; cover and simmer for about 10 minutes or until the orzo is almost done. Add a little more water or broth if needed.

Dice or pull the chicken into small pieces and stir into the skillet mixture. Stir in the peas and cook for 3 minutes more or until the orzo is done and the peas are cooked through. Turn off the heat and let sit covered for 3 minutes. Serve hot.

Nutritional Facts (per serving, about 1 1/2 cups):
Calories: 352
Carbohydrates: 45 g
Fiber: 6 g
Fat: 4.8 g
Sat. Fat: 0.8 g
Cholesterol: 53 mg
Protein: 30 g
Sodium: 432 mg
Calcium: 45 mg
Diabetic exchanges: 3 lean meat, 2 1/2 starch

Chicken Florentine
Yield: 4 servings

4 boneless skinless chicken breast halves (4 ounces each)
2 cups chicken broth
1/4 cup lemon juice
1/4 teaspoon ground black pepper
1 1/2 cup fresh or frozen whole kernel corn
3/4 cup thinly sliced leeks (white and light green parts only)
10 cups thinly sliced fresh spinach (10 ounces)
2 teaspoons cornstarch
1/3 cup nonfat or light sour cream

Place the chicken, broth, lemon juice, and pepper in a large nonstick skillet. Cover and cook over medium heat for several minutes, until the liquid begins to simmer. Adjust the heat to maintain a very low simmer. Cook for about 15 minutes or until the thickest part of the chicken reaches 165 degrees F. Remove the chicken to a small pot and add 1/2 cup of the poaching liquid. Cover and place on a back burner over low heat to keep warm.

Bring the poaching liquid that remains in the skillet to a boil. Cook uncovered for about 6 minutes to reduce the liquid to 1 cup. Pour 3/4 cup of the reduced liquid into a measuring cup and set aside.

Add the corn and leeks to the 1/4 cup of liquid remaining in the skillet. Cover and cook over medium heat for several minutes, until the leeks soften and the corn is cooked through. Add the spinach and cook uncovered for another minute or two, to wilt the spinach. Add a little water, if necessary, to prevent the skillet from drying out.

Divide the vegetable mixture between 4 serving plates. Thinly slice the chicken at an angle, and arrange a sliced chicken breast over the vegetables on each plate.

Mix the cornstarch with 2 teaspoons of water, and then stir into the reserved 3/4 cup of reduced broth. Pour the broth mixture into the skillet, and cook over medium heat, stirring frequently, for about a minute or until the broth comes to a boil and thickens slightly. Reduce the heat to low and whisk in the sour cream. Cook over low heat just to warm through (do not boil). Pour one-fourth of the sauce over each serving and serve immediately.

Nutritional Facts (per serving):
Calories: 228
Carbohydrates: 22 g
Fiber: 3.9 g
Fat: 2.2 g
Sat. Fat: 0.5 g
Cholesterol: 66 mg
Protein: 30 g
Sodium: 377 mg

Calcium: 127 mg

Diabetic exchanges: 3 lean meat, 1 starch, 1 vegetable

Chicken & Potato Pot Pie
Yield: 5 servings

10-ounce package frozen mixed vegetables
10 3/4-ounce can reduced-fat cream of celery soup, undiluted
3/4 cup nonfat or low-fat milk
2 cups diced poached chicken breast

TOPPING
3 cups diced Yukon Gold potatoes (leave on the peels for the most fiber)
2 garlic cloves
1/2 cup nonfat or light sour cream
1/4 teaspoon sea salt
Olive oil cooking spray
Ground paprika

Place the potatoes and garlic in a 2-quart pot. Add enough water to cover the potatoes and bring to a boil over medium heat. Cover and cook for about 10 minutes, stirring occasionally, until soft. Drain, reserving 1/3 cup of the cooking water. Return the potatoes and garlic cloves to the pot, add the sour cream and salt, and beat until smooth. Stir in just enough of the reserved cooking water to bring the potatoes to a creamy consistency.

While the potatoes are cooking, place the mixed vegetables and 1/2 cup of water in a 2-quart pot. Bring to a boil over medium heat. Cover and cook for 5 minutes, or until tender. Drain off the water, and add the undiluted soup and milk to the pot. Cook for a couple of minutes until the mixture comes to a boil. Stir in the chicken and heat through.

Coat a 9-inch deep-dish pie pan with cooking spray and spread the chicken mixture in the pan. Drop the potatoes in 5 mounds over the top. Spray the tops of the potatoes lightly with the cooking spray, and sprinkle lightly with paprika. Bake uncovered at 350 degrees for 20 to 25 minutes, or until bubbly around the edges. Serve hot.

Nutritional Facts (per serving):
Calories: 242
Carbohydrates: 32 g
Cholesterol: 47 mg
Fat: 3 g
Sat. Fat: 0.8 g
Fiber: 4.5 g
Protein: 24 g
Sodium: 454 mg
Calcium: 182 mg
Diabetic exchanges: 2 lean meat, 1 1/2 starch, 1 vegetable

Oven-Braised Turkey Breast
Yield: 6 servings

2 1/2-pound bone-in turkey breast half (remove the skin)
2 teaspoons crushed garlic
1 teaspoon dried herbes de Provence or fines herbes
3/4 teaspoon ground black pepper
3/4 teaspoon sea salt
1 cup dry white wine

GRAVY
1/2 cup nonfat or low-fat milk
3 tablespoons unbleached flour

Preheat the oven to 325 degrees F. Place the turkey breast, meaty side up, in a 9-by-13-inch pan. Combine the garlic, herbs, pepper, and salt and rub over the top of the meat. Pour the wine over and around the turkey breast. Cover the pan with aluminum foil and bake for 2 hours or until the meat is tender and cooked through. A thermometer inserted in the thickest part (not touching the bone) should read at least 165 degrees F. Let sit, covered loosely with foil, for 10 minutes.

To make the gravy, pour the pan juices into a 1-quart pot and place over medium heat. If necessary, boil uncovered for a few minutes to reduce the volume to 1 cup. Combine the milk and flour in a jar with a tight fitting lid and shake until smooth. Pour the flour mixture into the simmering broth, while stirring constantly. Cook for a minute or two until thickened and bubbly. Slice the turkey and serve with the gravy.

Nutritional Facts (per 3-ounce cooked turkey with 1/4 cup gravy)
Calories: 147
Carbohydrates: 4 g
Fiber: 0.3 g
Fat: 1 g
Sat. Fat: 0.3 g
Cholesterol: 59 mg
Protein: 23 g
Sodium: 408 mg
Calcium: 44 mg
Diabetic exchanges: 3 lean meat

Cajun Shrimp Boil
Yield: 4 servings

24 ounces beer (light or regular)
3 tablespoons Cajun or Creole seasoning
12 ounces red-skinned new potatoes (about 6 medium), cut into 1 1/2-inch pieces
3 medium ears fresh shucked corn, each cut into 3 pieces
2 1/2 cups fresh broccoli or cauliflower florets (2-inch pieces)
1 1/4 pounds large raw unpeeled shrimp

Pour the beer into a 6-quart pot and add enough water to half fill the pot. Add the Cajun seasoning and potatoes and bring to a boil. Boil covered, with the lid slightly ajar, for 5 minutes. Add the corn and boil for 4 minutes or until the potatoes and corn are nearly done. Add the broccoli or cauliflower and boil for 1 minute.

Add the shrimp and boil for 2 to 3 minutes more or just until the shrimp turn opaque and are cooked through. Drain well and serve hot.

Nutritional Facts (per serving):
Calories: 213
Carbohydrates: 30 g
Fiber: 4.9 g
Fat: 1.9 g
Sat. Fat: 0.4 g
Cholesterol: 168 mg
Protein: 24 g
Sodium: 515 mg
Calcium: 68 mg
Diabetic exchanges: 3 lean meat, 1 1/2 starch, 1 vegetable

Steamed Fish with Ginger Sauce
Yield: 2 servings

1 green tea bag
5 thin slices fresh ginger
2 large leaves napa or Chinese cabbage
2 whitefish fillets (such as tilapia or cod) or salmon fillets (4 to 5 ounces each)
1/3 cup thinly sliced leek (white and light green parts)
1/2 cup matchstick carrots
2 teaspoons reduced-sodium soy sauce

SAUCE
1 tablespoon reduced-sodium soy sauce

1 teaspoon finely grated fresh ginger
1/2 teaspoon canola or non-toasted sesame oil

Combine the sauce ingredients in a small bowl and set aside.

Cut the tea bag open and pour the leaves into a 6-quart pot; add the ginger slices. Add a steamer basket and fill with enough water to reach within 1/2 inch of the bottom of the basket. Place the cabbage leaves on the steamer and arrange the fish fillets over the leaves. Sprinkle half of the leeks and carrots over each fish fillet. Drizzle each fillet with 1 teaspoon of soy sauce.

Cover the pot and bring to a boil. Let the fish steam for about 10 minutes or until it flakes easily with a fork. Use a spatula to remove the cabbage and fish to serving plates. Stir the sauce and drizzle half over each fish fillet. Serve immediately.

Nutritional Facts (per serving):
Calories: 138
Carbohydrates: 6 g
Fiber: 0.7 g
Fat: 3.2 g
Sat. Fat: 0.8 g
Cholesterol: 54 mg
Protein: 23 g
Sodium: 417 mg
Calcium: 40 mg
Diabetic exchanges: 3 lean meat, 1 vegetable

Mediterranean Baked Fish
Yield: 4 servings

1 fresh lemon, thinly sliced
4 white fish fillets such as cod or tilapia (4 to 5 ounces each)
1 1/2 teaspoons crushed garlic
3/4 teaspoon dried oregano
scant 1/2 teaspoon sea salt

1/2 teaspoon ground black pepper
2 medium plum tomatoes, thinly sliced
1 medium yellow onion, thinly sliced
1/2 cup finely chopped fresh parsley
1/4 cup white wine
1 1/2 tablespoons extra virgin olive oil

Preheat the oven to 400 degrees F. Coat a baking pan (large enough to hold the fish fillets in a single layer) with cooking spray and lay the lemon slices over the bottom of the pan. Place the fish over the lemon slices and sprinkle with the garlic, oregano, and half of the salt and pepper. Layer on the tomato slices, and sprinkle with the remaining salt and pepper. Top with the onion and parsley. Pour the wine over the top and drizzle with the olive oil.

Cover the pan with foil and bake for 20 minutes, until the fish flakes easily. Serve over whole wheat orzo, couscous, or angel hair pasta if desired.

Nutritional Facts:
Calories: 170
Carbohydrates: 6 g
Fiber: 1.3 g
Fat: 6.3 g
Sat. Fat: 1.2 g
Cholesterol: 54 mg
Protein: 22 g
Sodium: 324 mg
Calcium: 47 mg
Diabetic exchanges: 3 lean meat, 1 vegetable

Foil-Baked Fish with Summer Vegetables
Yield: 4 servings

1 cup fresh or frozen (thawed) whole kernel corn
1 cup diced zucchini

1 cup quartered grape or cherry tomatoes
6 thin slices yellow onion, cut into quarter-rings
1/2 teaspoon ground black pepper
1/4 teaspoon sea salt
1 teaspoon dried thyme, dill, or marjoram
4 pieces of aluminum foil (12-inch squares) or parchment paper (15-inch squares)
4 flounder, tilapia, cod, or other white fish fillets (4 to 5 ounces each)
4 teaspoons extra virgin olive oil

Preheat the oven to 400 degrees F. Place the corn, zucchini, tomatoes, and onion in a bowl. Add half of the pepper, salt, and herbs and toss to mix. Set aside.

Lay a fish fillet on the lower part of each piece of foil or parchment. Sprinkle the fillets with the remaining pepper, salt, and herbs. Top each fillet with one-fourth of the vegetable mixture. Fold the top part of the foil or parchment over the lower part to enclose the fish and vegetables. Double-fold the edges together to tightly seal the packets.

Lay the packets on a large baking sheet and bake for 20 minutes, until the fish is cooked through and flakes easily. Open with care, as steam will escape. Serve hot, drizzling a teaspoon of the olive oil over each serving.

Nutritional Facts (per serving):
Calories: 179
Carbohydrates: 12 g
Fiber: 1.8 g
Fat: 6 g
Sat. Fat: 1.2 g
Cholesterol: 54 mg
Protein: 23 g
Sodium: 220 mg
Calcium: 33 mg
Diabetic exchanges: 3 lean meat, 1/2 starch, 1 vegetable

Foil-Baked Fish with Asparagus, Orange, & Onion
Yield: 4 servings

4 pieces of aluminum foil (12-inch squares) or parchment paper (15-inch squares)
4 fish fillets such as cod, halibut, or salmon (5 ounces each)
1/4 teaspoon sea salt
1/4 teaspoon ground black pepper
3/4 teaspoon dried tarragon or fines herbes or 2 1/2 teaspoons fresh
4 thin slices sweet white onion, separated into rings
2 1/2 cups 1 1/2-inch pieces fresh asparagus spears
4 tablespoons orange juice
1 tablespoon extra virgin olive oil

Preheat the oven to 400 degrees F. Place one fish fillet over the bottom half of each piece of foil or parchment and sprinkle with one-fourth of the salt, pepper, and tarragon or fines herbs. Top each fillet with one-fourth of the onion slices and asparagus and drizzle with 1 tablespoon of the orange juice.

Fold the top part of the foil or parchment over the lower part to enclose the fish and vegetables. Double-fold the edges together to tightly seal the packets. Lay the packets on a large baking sheet and bake for 20 minutes, until the fish is cooked through and flakes easily.

Carefully cut the packets open (steam will escape) and drizzle some of the olive oil over each serving. Serve over brown rice or whole wheat couscous if desired.

Nutritional Facts (per serving):
Calories: 206
Carbohydrates: 12 g
Fiber: 3.7 g
Fat: 4.6 g
Sat. Fat: 0.7 g
Cholesterol: 61 mg

Protein: 29 g

Sodium: 368 mg

Calcium: 66 mg

Diabetic exchanges: 4 lean meat, 1 1/2 vegetable

Whitefish with Tomatoes, Peas & Parsley Sauce
Yield: 2 servings

3-4 lemon slices
3/4 teaspoon whole peppercorns or scant 1/2 teaspoon ground black pepper
2 whitefish fillets such as halibut or cod (4 ounces each)
1 medium fresh tomato, chopped
1 cup frozen green peas, thawed
1/2 cup chopped sweet white or red onion
1 teaspoon capers
1 1/2 cups fresh arugula

SAUCE
1 tablespoon very finely chopped fresh parsley
1 tablespoon extra virgin olive oil
1 clove fresh garlic, crushed
Juice of one fresh lemon
1/8 teaspoon sea salt

Pour 1 inch of water into a 6-quart pot. Add the lemon slices and pepper to the water and then place a steamer basket in the pot. Arrange the fish fillets in a single layer in the basket. Cover and bring to a boil. Let the fish steam for about 10 minutes or until it flakes easily with a fork.

Place the fish in a bowl and add the tomatoes, peas, onion, and capers. Gently toss the mixture, allowing the fish to flake into chunks. Arrange half the arugula leaves on each of two serving plates and top each serving with half of the fish mixture. Combine the sauce ingredients, stir to mix, and drizzle over the top. Serve immediately.

Nutritional Facts (per serving):

Calories: 275

Carbohydrates: 18 g

Fiber: 5.1 g

Fat: 9.9 g

Sat. Fat: 1.4 g

Cholesterol: 36 mg

Protein: 29 g

Sodium: 339 mg

Calcium: 101 mg

Diabetic exchanges: 3 lean meat, 1/2 starch, 1 1/2 vegetable, 1 1/2 fat

Cod with Tomatoes & Capers

Yield: 4 servings

4 pieces of aluminum foil (12-inch squares) or parchment paper (15-inch squares)

8 to 12 thin slices fresh lemon

4 cod, tilapia, or other whitefish fillets (4 to 5 ounces each)

1 teaspoon crushed garlic

1/2 teaspoon ground black pepper

1/4 teaspoon sea salt

3/4 teaspoon dried thyme or oregano or 2 1/2 teaspoons fresh

1 cup quartered grape or cherry tomatoes

1/2 cup thinly sliced leek (white and light green parts)

4 teaspoons capers, drained

4 teaspoons extra virgin olive oil

Preheat the oven to 400 degrees F. Lay 2 or 3 lemon slices on the lower part of each piece of foil or parchment and top with a fish fillet. Sprinkle the fillets with one-fourth of the garlic, pepper, salt, and thyme or oregano. Top each fillet with one-fourth of the tomatoes, leeks, and capers.

Fold the top part of the foil or parchment over the lower part to enclose the fish and vegetables. Double-fold the edges together to tightly seal the packets. Lay the packets on a large baking sheet and bake for 20 minutes, until the fish flakes easily. Open with care, as steam will escape. Serve hot, drizzling a teaspoon of the olive oil over each serving. Serve over whole wheat couscous, orzo, or angel hair pasta if desired.

Nutritional Facts (per serving):
Calories: 152
Carbohydrates: 5 g
Fiber: 1 g
Fat: 5.5 g
Sat. Fat: 0.8 g
Cholesterol: 48 mg
Protein: 21 g
Sodium: 297 mg
Calcium: 34 mg
Diabetic exchanges: 3 lean meat, 1 fat

Pasta with Shrimp & Scallops Arrabbiata
Yield: 5 servings

2 tablespoons olive oil
2 teaspoons crushed garlic
28-ounce can crushed tomatoes
1/4 cup vegetable broth or white wine
1/2 teaspoon crushed red pepper
1/2 cup finely chopped fresh parsley
8 ounces peeled and deveined raw shrimp
8 ounces raw scallops
10 ounces whole grain penne pasta, cooked al dente and drained

Place 1 tablespoon of the olive oil and all of the garlic in a large deep skillet and place over medium heat. Cook for about 30 seconds or just until the garlic begins to turn color and smells fragrant. Add the tomatoes, broth or wine, red pepper, and half of the parsley and bring to a boil. Reduce the heat to maintain a simmer; cover and cook for 15 minutes.

Increase the heat to medium and add the shrimp and scallops. Let the mixture come to a boil and cook with the cover on, stirring frequently, for about 3 minutes or until the seafood turns opaque and is cooked through. Stir in the remaining olive oil. Add the pasta and the remaining parsley to the skillet and toss to mix. Serve hot.

Nutritional Facts (per 2 1/4-cup serving):
Calories: 368
Carbohydrates: 50 g
Fiber: 6.8 g
Fat: 7.5 g
Sat. Fat: 1.1 g
Cholesterol: 84 mg
Protein: 27 g
Sodium: 438 mg
Calcium: 118 mg
Diabetic exchanges: 2 1/2 starch, 2 vegetable, 2 1/2 lean meat

Pasta with Shrimp & Broccoli
Yield: 5 servings

8 ounces whole grain penne or rotini pasta
4 cups fresh broccoli florets
3 tablespoons extra virgin olive oil
1 medium yellow onion, cut into thin wedges
2 teaspoons crushed garlic
1 cup dry white wine
1 pound peeled and deveined raw shrimp
1/2 teaspoon sea salt
1/2 teaspoon ground black pepper
1 tablespoon plus 1 teaspoon grated Parmesan cheese
1 tablespoon finely chopped fresh oregano or 1 teaspoon dried

Cook the pasta according to package directions. Two minutes before the pasta is done, add the broccoli to the pot and cook until the broccoli is crisp-tender and the pasta is done. Drain the pasta and broccoli and set aside to keep warm.

While the pasta is cooking, place 1 tablespoon of the olive oil and all of the onion in a large deep nonstick skillet. Cover and cook over medium heat for several minutes, until the onion starts to soften (add a little water if needed to prevent scorching). Add the garlic and cook for about 15 seconds. Add the wine and adjust the heat to maintain a simmer. Cover and cook for 3 minutes.

Add the shrimp, salt, and pepper to the skillet and increase the heat to medium. Cook uncovered for about 3 minutes, stirring occasionally, until the shrimp turn opaque and are cooked through. Add the pasta, broccoli, and remaining olive oil and toss to heat through. Remove from the heat and toss in the Parmesan. Sprinkle with the oregano and serve immediately.

Nutritional Facts (per 2-cup serving):
Calories: 375
Carbohydrates: 37 g
Fiber: 5.3 g
Fat: 10.9 g
Sat. Fat: 1.8 g
Cholesterol: 139 mg
Protein: 27 g
Sodium: 420 mg
Calcium: 123 mg
Diabetic exchanges: 2 starch, 1 vegetable, 2 1/2 lean meat, 1 1/2 fat

Penne with Spicy Shrimp & Artichokes
Yield: 5 servings

2 tablespoons extra virgin olive oil
1 medium yellow onion, cut into thin wedges
2 teaspoons crushed garlic

2 cans (14 1/2 ounces each) diced tomatoes with celery, green peppers, and onion, non-drained
1/4 cup dry white wine
1 1/2 tablespoons finely chopped fresh basil or 1 1/2 teaspoons dried basil
1/2 teaspoon dried oregano
1/4 teaspoon ground black pepper
1/4 teaspoon crushed red pepper
1 pound peeled and deveined raw shrimp
15-ounce can artichoke hearts, drained and coarsely chopped
1/3 cup sliced black olives
8 ounces whole grain penne pasta, cooked al dente

Place 1 tablespoon of the olive oil and all of the onion in a large, deep nonstick skillet. Add 1 tablespoon of water and place over medium heat. Cover and cook for several minutes, stirring occasionally, until the onion softens. Add a little water, if needed, to prevent scorching. Stir in the garlic and cook for about 15 seconds. Add the tomatoes, wine, basil, oregano, black pepper, and red pepper and bring to a boil. Reduce the heat to maintain a simmer; cover and cook for 3 minutes.

Add the shrimp to the skillet mixture and bring to a boil. Reduce the heat to medium, cover, and cook for about 3 minutes, or just until the shrimp turn opaque and are cooked through. Add the artichoke hearts and olives and cook for about a minute to heat through.

Add the pasta and remaining olive oil and toss over low heat for a minute or two to heat through. Serve hot.

Nutritional Facts (per 2 1/4-cup serving):
Calories: 387
Carbohydrates: 49 g
Fiber: 8.4 g
Fat: 8.6 g
Sat. Fat: 1.3 g
Cholesterol: 138 mg
Protein: 28 g

Sodium: 886 mg

Calcium: 134 mg

Diabetic exchanges: 2 starch, 2 vegetable, 2 1/2 lean meat, 1 fat

Crab Cakes with Roasted Red Pepper Sauce
Yield: 5 servings

2/3 cup finely chopped red bell pepper
1/3 cup finely chopped scallions
1 teaspoon crushed garlic
1 pound lump crabmeat, picked over to remove any shell pieces
2 tablespoons nonfat or low-fat mayonnaise
1 to 2 teaspoons Cajun seasoning
2 tablespoons fat-free egg substitute or 1 egg white, beaten
1/2 cup soft-textured oat bran
Olive oil cooking spray

SAUCE
1/2 cup jarred roasted red bell peppers, drained and chopped
1/2 cup nonfat mayonnaise
1 tablespoon extra virgin olive oil
1 teaspoon crushed garlic
1/4 teaspoon ground black pepper
1/8 teaspoon cayenne pepper (optional)

To make the sauce, combine all of the sauce ingredients in a mini food processor and process until smooth. Cover and chill until ready to serve.

Coat a medium nonstick skillet with cooking spray. Add the bell pepper and scallions, and place over medium heat. Cover and cook for several minutes, stirring occasionally, until soft. Add a few teaspoons of water during cooking if needed to prevent scorching. Add the garlic and cook for about 15 seconds. Remove from the heat and set aside.

Place the crabmeat in a large bowl and add the mayonnaise, Cajun seasoning, egg substitute or egg white, and 2 tablespoons of the oat bran. Add the sautéed vegetables and toss to mix. Place the remaining oat bran in a shallow container. Shape a scant 1/3 cup portion of the crab mixture into a ball and flatten into a 1/2-inch thick patty. Dip in the oat bran, coating both sides. Repeat to make 10 patties, and place the patties in a single layer on a baking sheet. Cover and chill for at least 1 hour.

Coat a large nonstick skillet with cooking spray and preheat over medium heat until a drop of water sizzles when added. Spray the tops of the patties lightly with the cooking spray, and add half of the patties, sprayed side up, to the skillet. Cover and cook for 3 minutes. Turn the patties over and cook for 3 minutes more or, until golden brown and cooked through. Wipe out and re-spray the skillet; then cook the remaining crab cakes. Serve hot.

Nutritional Facts (per serving, 2 cakes):
Calories: 177
Carbohydrates: 16 g
Fiber: 2.2 g
Fat: 5.1 g
Sat. Fat: 0.7 g
Cholesterol: 91 mg
Protein: 21 g
Sodium: 572 mg
Calcium: 112 mg
Diabetic exchanges: 3 lean meat, 1 starch

Ceviche*
Yield: 4 servings

1 pound very fresh, raw bay (small) scallops
8 limes, juiced
2 medium tomatoes, diced
5 scallions, finely chopped
2 stalks celery, thinly sliced

1/2 green bell pepper, finely chopped
1/2 cup chopped fresh parsley
2 tablespoons chopped fresh cilantro
1 1/2 tablespoons olive oil
Freshly ground black pepper

Rinse the scallops and place in a medium sized bowl. Pour the lime juice over the scallops. The scallops should be completely immersed in the lime juice. Chill the lime juice and scallops all day or overnight until scallops are opaque.

Empty half of the lime juice from the bowl. Add the tomatoes, scallions, celery, green bell pepper, parsley, cilantro, olive oil, and black pepper to the scallop mixture. Stir gently. Serve this dish in fancy glasses with a slice of lime hanging over the rim for garnish.

Nutritional Facts (per serving):
Calories: 182
Carbohydrates: 12 g
Fiber: 2.1 g
Fat: 6.3 g
Sat. Fat: 0.8 g
Cholesterol: 37 mg
Protein: 20 g
Sodium: 213 mg
Calcium: 62 mg
Diabetic exchanges: 3 lean meat, 1 1/2 vegetable

*Note that ceviche is not cooked, so it should be avoided by those who have been advised not to eat raw seafood.

Flavorful Fried Rice
Yield: 4 servings

1/2 cup fat-free egg substitute or 2 eggs, beaten
1 tablespoon canola oil
2 to 3 cups thinly sliced Chinese cabbage, bok choy, or green cabbage

1 cup sliced scallions
1/4 cup vegetable or chicken broth
2 to 3 teaspoons finely grated fresh ginger
1 1/2 teaspoons crushed garlic
1 cup cooked shelled edamame or frozen green peas (thawed)
3 cups cooked brown rice
3 to 4 tablespoons reduced-sodium soy sauce
1 cup steamed or boiled shrimp, chopped poached chicken, or cubed extra-firm tofu

Coat a large nonstick skillet with cooking spray and preheat over medium heat until a drop of water sizzles when added. Pour the eggs into the skillet and swirl to evenly coat the bottom of the pan. Cook without stirring for a couple of minutes, or until firm. Slide the eggs onto a large cutting board, slice into thin strips, and set aside.

Pour the oil into the skillet and add the cabbage, scallions, and broth. Cover and cook for several minutes, until the cabbage is wilted and tender. Add the ginger and garlic and cook for 15 seconds more. Stir in the edamame or peas and cook with the cover on for another minute to heat through.

Add the rice, soy sauce, eggs, and the shrimp, chicken, or tofu. Cover and cook for a couple of minutes, stirring occasionally, until heated through.

Nutritional Facts (per serving, about 1 1/2 cups):
Calories: 323
Carbohydrate: 42 g
Fiber: 6 g
Fat: 8.1 g
Sat. Fat: 1 g
Cholesterol: 69 mg
Protein: 21 g
Sodium: 665 mg
Calcium: 125 mg
Diabetic exchanges: 2 lean meat, 2 1/2 starch, 1 vegetable, 1/2 fat

For variety: Add 1 cup fresh Chinese mushrooms, sliced white button mushrooms, or small broccoli florets along with the cabbage.

Cajun Meatloaf
Yield: 6 servings

1 1/2 cups sliced fresh mushrooms
1/3 cup chopped onion
1/3 cup chopped green bell pepper
1 1/4 pounds ground beef (at least 93% lean)
1/2 cup quick-cooking (1-minute) oats
1 tablespoon plus 1 teaspoon Dijon mustard
1 tablespoon plus 1 teaspoon dried parsley
1/2 teaspoon ground black pepper
1 1/2 teaspoons Cajun seasoning, divided
8-ounce can no-added-salt tomato sauce

Preheat the oven to 350 degrees F. Place the mushrooms, onion, and bell pepper in a food processor and process until very finely chopped. Transfer to a large bowl. Add the ground meat, oats, mustard, parsley, black pepper, and 1 teaspoon of the Cajun seasoning and mix well. Coat a 9-by-5-inch meatloaf pan with cooking spray and press the mixture into the pan.

Stir the remaining Cajun seasoning into the tomato sauce and spread the tomato sauce over the top of the meatloaf. Bake uncovered for 1 hour or until done (a meat thermometer inserted in the center of the loaf should read at least 160 degrees F). Let sit for 10 minutes before slicing and serving.

Nutritional Facts (per serving):
Calories: 198
Carbohydrates: 10 g
Fiber: 2 g
Fat: 7.5 g

Sat. Fat: 2.9 g

Cholesterol: 59 mg

Protein: 22 g

Sodium: 272 mg

Calcium: 30 mg

Diabetic exchanges: 3 lean meat, 1/2 carbohydrate

Spaghetti & Meatballs
Yield: 5 servings

1 ounce firm whole grain bread (about 1 slice)
1 1/2 cups sliced fresh mushrooms
1 pound ground beef (at least 93% lean)
1/4 cup finely chopped fresh parsley or 4 teaspoons dried
2 tablespoons finely chopped fresh basil or 2 teaspoons dried
1 teaspoon crushed garlic
1/2 teaspoon ground black pepper
1 egg white, beaten or 2 tablespoons fat-free egg substitute
3 cups ready-made low-fat marinara sauce
1/2 cup low-sodium vegetable or beef broth
10 ounces whole grain spaghetti or penne pasta, cooked al dente

Tear the bread into chunks, place in a food processor, and process into crumbs. Transfer the crumbs to a large bowl. Add the mushrooms to the food processor and finely chop. Add the mushrooms to the bowl with the breadcrumbs. Add the ground meat, parsley, basil, garlic, pepper, and egg white to the breadcrumbs and mushrooms, and mix well. Shape the mixture into 15 meatballs, each about 1 3/4 inches in diameter. Set aside.

Pour the marinara sauce and broth into a large deep nonstick skillet and bring to a boil over medium heat. Add the meatballs to the skillet and reduce the heat to maintain a simmer. Cover and simmer for 30 to 40 minutes, turning the meatballs and stirring occasionally. If necessary, simmer uncovered for a few minutes to allow the sauce to thicken a bit. Serve hot over the pasta.

Nutritional Facts (per serving):
Calories: 393
Carbohydrates: 52 g
Fiber: 9.4 g
Fat: 8.6 g
Sat. Fat: 2.9 g
Cholesterol: 57 mg
Protein: 31 g
Sodium: 735 mg
Calcium: 67 mg
Diabetic exchanges: 2 1/2 lean meat, 3 starch, 1 vegetable

Variation:

To make Meatball Sandwiches, place 3 meatballs with some of the sauce in a 4-inch whole grain sub roll or baguette. Top with 2 tablespoons shredded reduced-fat mozzarella cheese.

Oven Braised Pot Roast
Yield: 6 servings

2 1/4-pound well-trimmed top round roast
1/2 cup dry red wine
1/2 cup beef broth
2 teaspoons crushed garlic
1 teaspoon dried rosemary
1 teaspoon dried thyme
1/2 teaspoon sea salt
1/2 teaspoon ground black pepper

GRAVY
1/2 teaspoon beef bouillon granules
3 tablespoons whole wheat pastry flour or unbleached flour
1/4 cup water

Preheat the oven to 300 degrees F. Coat a large deep ovenproof skillet with cooking spray and preheat over medium heat. Add the roast and cook for about 2 minutes on each side to lightly brown and seal the meat. Remove the skillet from heat.

Combine the wine, broth, garlic, rosemary, thyme, salt, and pepper and pour over the roast. Cover the skillet tightly with aluminum foil and bake for about 3 hours, or until the roast is very tender and can be easily pulled apart with a fork. Remove the roast from the oven and transfer to a large cutting board (caution: steam will escape). Cover loosely with foil and let sit for 10 minutes.

To make the gravy, pour the pan juices into a 2-quart pot and add the bouillon granules. Place over medium heat and boil until reduced to 1 1/4 cups. Combine the flour and water in a small jar with a tight-fitting lid and shake until smooth. Slowly pour the flour mixture into the simmering broth. Cook and stir for a couple of minutes, until thickened. Slice the roast and serve with the gravy.

Nutritional Facts (per 3-oz. cooked meat with 1/4 cup gravy):

Calories: 208

Carbohydrates: 4 g

Fiber: 0.7 g

Fat: 5.5 g

Sat. Fat: 1.9 g

Cholesterol: 76 mg

Protein: 31 g

Sodium: 373 mg

Calcium: 10 mg

Diabetic exchanges: 3 lean meat

Chili-Macaroni

Yield: 6 servings

1 pound ground beef (at least 93% lean)
1 medium yellow onion, chopped
14 1/2-ounce can Mexican-style diced tomatoes, non-drained and crushed

15-ounce can dark red kidney beans, drained
1 1/4 cups beef broth
1 1/4 cups V-8 vegetable juice
1 tablespoon chili powder
1 teaspoon ground cumin
1/2 teaspoon dried oregano
6 ounces uncooked whole grain elbow or ziti macaroni

Coat a large deep nonstick skillet with cooking spray and add the ground meat and onion. Place over medium heat, cover, and cook for about 6 minutes, stirring to crumble, until the meat is no longer pink (do not drain). Add the non-drained tomatoes, beans, broth, V-8 juice, chili powder, cumin, and oregano and bring to a boil.

Add the macaroni to the skillet and stir to mix. Reduce the heat to medium; cover and cook for about 10 minutes or until most of the liquid is absorbed and the macaroni is tender. Stir occasionally. Add a little more V-8 juice or broth if needed. Serve hot.

Nutritional Facts (per 1 1/2-cup serving):
Calories: 334
Carbohydrates: 45 g
Fiber: 10 g
Fat: 6.3 g
Sat fat: 2.4 g
Cholesterol: 47 mg
Protein: 26 g
Sodium: 591 mg
Calcium: 50 mg
Diabetic exchanges: 2 1/2 lean meat, 2 1/2 starch, 1 vegetable

Greek-Style Skillet Dinner
Yield: 4 servings

3/4 pound ground beef or lamb (at least 93% lean)
1 cup chopped yellow onion

3/4 cup chopped carrot (1/4-inch dice)
2 teaspoons crushed garlic
1 teaspoon dried oregano
1/4 teaspoon ground cinnamon
2 1/4 cups beef broth
1 cup V-8 vegetable juice
1/4 teaspoon ground black pepper
1 cup uncooked quick-cooking barley or whole wheat orzo
1/4 cup finely chopped fresh parsley
2 tablespoons finely chopped fresh mint
1 1/2 teaspoons lemon juice

Coat a large nonstick skillet with cooking spray and add the ground meat and onion. Cover and cook over medium heat for about 6 minutes, stirring to crumble, until the meat is no longer pink (do not drain). Add the carrots, garlic, oregano, cinnamon, and 1 cup of the broth. Cover and cook over medium heat for 5 minutes or until the carrots start to soften.

Add the remaining broth and the V-8 juice, pepper, and barley or orzo. Cover and cook over medium heat for about 15 minutes or until the barley or orzo is tender. Add a little more broth if the mixture seems too dry. Stir in the parsley, mint, and lemon juice. Turn off the heat and let sit covered for 5 minutes before serving.

Nutritional Facts (per 1 1/2-cup serving):
Calories: 297
Carbohydrates: 37 g
Fiber: 6 g
Fat: 7 g
Sat fat: 2.7 g
Cholesterol: 53 mg
Protein: 23 g
Sodium: 637 mg
Calcium: 522 mg
Diabetic exchanges: 2 1/2 lean meat, 2 starch, 1 1/2 vegetable

Skillet Beef Stroganoff
Yield: 4 servings

3/4 pound ground beef (at least 93% lean)
2 1/2 cups sliced fresh mushrooms
1/2 cup finely chopped yellow onion
2 cups beef broth
1/2 cup plus 2 tablespoons V-8 vegetable juice
Scant 1/2 teaspoon ground black pepper
6 ounces whole grain noodles
1 cup nonfat or light sour cream
3/4 teaspoon Dijon mustard

Coat a large deep skillet with cooking spray and add the ground beef, mushrooms, and onion. Cover and cook over medium heat for about 6 minutes, stirring to crumble, until the meat is no longer pink (do not drain).

Add the broth, vegetable juice, and pepper to the skillet and bring to a boil. Stir in the noodles and reduce the heat to medium. Cover and cook for about 10 minutes, stirring occasionally, or until most of the liquid has been absorbed and the noodles are tender. Add a little more broth if needed to keep about 1/4 cup of liquid in the skillet.

Reduce the heat to low. Stir the mustard into the sour cream and then gently stir the sour cream mixture into the skillet. Cook and stir for about a minute to warm through (do not boil). Serve hot.

Nutritional Facts (per 1 3/4-cup serving)
Calories: 332
Carbohydrates: 40 g
Fiber: 4 g
Fat: 6.8 g
Sat. Fat: 2.7 g
Cholesterol: 53 mg
Protein: 27 g

Sodium: 671 mg

Calcium: 121 mg

Diabetic exchanges: 2 1/2 lean meat, 2 1/2 starch, 1 vegetable

Saucy Stuffed Cabbage
Yield: 5 servings

1 1/2 cups chopped yellow onion
1/2 cup grated carrot
3 tablespoons water
1 teaspoon dried thyme
2 teaspoons crushed garlic
3/4 cup uncooked bulgur wheat or whole wheat orzo
1/2 teaspoon sea salt
1/2 teaspoon ground black pepper
1 pound ground beef (at least 93% lean)
8 large cabbage or collard leaves (each about 8 inches wide by 8 to 10 inches long)

SAUCE
14 1/2-ounce can stewed tomatoes or diced tomatoes with green peppers and onions, non-drained
1 cup beef broth
1 tablespoon dark brown sugar
1 tablespoon apple cider vinegar
1/2 teaspoon ground cinnamon
1 tablespoon unbleached flour

Preheat the oven to 350 degrees F. Coat a large nonstick skillet with cooking spray and add the onion, carrot, water, and thyme. Cover and cook over medium heat for about 6 minutes or until the vegetables soften. Stir in the garlic and cook for 15 seconds more. Remove from the heat and stir in the bulgur wheat or orzo, salt, and pepper. Set aside.

Place all of the sauce ingredients except for the flour in a blender and puree until smooth. Stir 1/2 cup of the pureed tomato mixture into the skillet mixture. Add the beef and mix well. Set aside.

Cut the cabbage or collard leaves in half along the tough center vein, trimming away the vein and discarding it. Place 1/4 cup (packed) of the beef mixture along the bottom of a cabbage or collard half-leaf and roll the leaf up to enclose the filling. Continue in this manner to make 15 filled leaves. Spray a 10-by-13-inch pan with cooking spray and arrange the rolls in a single layer in the pan, seam side down.

Add the flour to the pureed tomatoes remaining in the blender and blend until smooth. Pour into a 2-quart pot and bring to a boil, stirring frequently. Pour the sauce over the cabbage rolls. Cover the pan with aluminum foil and bake for 45 minutes or until the filling is firm and the grain is cooked. The filling should reach at least 160 degrees F. Let sit for 5 minutes before serving.

Nutritional Facts (per serving):
Calories: 283
Carbohydrates: 33 g
Fiber: 7.3 g
Fat: 6.8 g
Sat. Fat: 2.8 g
Cholesterol: 57 mg
Protein: 23 g
Sodium: 712 mg
Calcium: 64 mg
Diabetic exchanges: 2 1/2 lean meat, 2 carbohydrate

Soft Tacos
Yield: 10 tacos

10-ounce can Rotelle tomatoes with green chilies, non-drained
1 teaspoon chili powder
1/2 teaspoon ground cumin

1/2 teaspoon dried oregano
1 pound ground beef, chicken, turkey (at least 93% lean)
3/4 cup chopped yellow onion
10 corn or whole grain flour tortillas (6-inch rounds)

TOPPINGS
1/2 cup nonfat or light sour cream
1/2 cup shredded reduced-fat cheddar or Monterey Jack cheese
1 1/2 cups shredded lettuce

Place the tomatoes, chili powder, cumin, and oregano in a blender and blend until smooth. Set aside. Coat a large nonstick skillet with cooking spray and add the ground meat and onion. Cover and cook over medium heat for about 6 minutes, stirring to crumble, until the meat is no longer pink (do not drain).

Add the blended tomato mixture to the skillet and stir to mix. Cover and cook for 3 minutes. Remove the lid and cook for a couple of minutes more, or until most of the liquid has evaporated. Set aside to keep warm.

Heat the tortillas according to package directions. Fill each tortilla with about 1/4 cup of the meat mixture, and about 2 1/2 teaspoons each of sour cream and cheese. Top with some of the lettuce. Serve hot.

Nutritional Facts (per 2 tacos):
Calories: 286
Carbohydrates: 24 g
Fiber: 3.5 g
Fat: 9.3 g
Sat fat: 3.9 g
Cholesterol: 63 mg
Protein: 26 g
Sodium: 418 mg
Calcium: 166 mg
Diabetic exchanges: 3 lean meat, 1 1/2 starch, 1 vegetable

Pork Carnitas
Yield: 8 servings

2 teaspoons crushed garlic
2 teaspoons dried oregano
1 teaspoon ground cumin
1 1/2 teaspoons ground black pepper
1 teaspoon sea salt
2 1/4 pound well-trimmed pork loin or sirloin roast
1 cup beer (light or regular)

Preheat the oven to 325 degrees F. Combine the garlic, oregano, cumin, pepper, and salt and stir to mix. Rub over all sides of the roast. Coat a 9-by-13-inch pan with cooking spray and lay the roast in the pan. Pour the beer around the roast.

Cover the pan with aluminum foil and bake for 2 1/2 hours or until the roast can be easily pulled apart with a fork. Remove from the oven and let sit, covered loosely with foil for 10 minutes. Pull the meat into chunks and toss in some of the cooking liquid to moisten. Serve with warm corn tortillas, salsa, and avocado slices or spoon over brown rice or quinoa and sprinkle with some fresh chopped cilantro or fresh tomato salsa.

Nutritional Facts (per 3-ounce serving, meat only):
Calories: 171
Carbohydrates: 1 g
Fiber: 0.3 g
Fat: 4.6 g
Sat fat: 1.7 g
Cholesterol: 74 mg
Protein: 26 g
Sodium: 369 mg
Calcium: 11 mg
Diabetic exchanges: 3 lean meat

Pork Tenderloin with Sour Cream Sauce
Yield: 4 servings

1 pound pork tenderloin
1 teaspoon dried sage
1/4 teaspoon ground black pepper
1/4 teaspoon sea salt
1/2 cup chicken broth
1/2 cup dry white wine
1 teaspoon crushed garlic
1/4 cup nonfat or light sour cream
1 teaspoon Dijon mustard
1 tablespoon cornstarch
2 tablespoons finely chopped fresh parsley or 2 teaspoons dried

Rub the tenderloin all over with the sage, pepper, and salt. Coat a large skillet with cooking spray and preheat over medium heat. Add the pork and cook for a minute or two, just enough to lightly brown and seal the meat on all sides. Add the broth, wine, and garlic to the skillet and reduce the heat to maintain a simmer. Cover and cook, turning occasionally, for about 20 minutes or until a thermometer inserted in the thickest part registers at least 155 degrees F. Remove the pork and set aside to keep warm.

To make the sauce, combine the sour cream and mustard and stir to mix. Set aside. Measure the liquid in the skillet and, if necessary, cook uncovered for a few minutes to reduce to 3/4 cup in volume. Combine the cornstarch with 1 tablespoon of water and stir to dissolve; whisk into the liquid in the skillet. Simmer for a minute or two until thickened and bubbly. Reduce the heat to low and whisk in the sour cream mixture. Remove from the heat.

To serve, thinly slice the pork at an angle and divide the slices between 4 plates. Drizzle some of the sauce over each serving and top with a sprinkling of parsley.

Nutritional Facts (per serving):

Calories: 195

Carbohydrates: 4 g

Fiber: 0.2 g

Fat: 6.3 g

Sat. Fat: 2.1 g

Cholesterol: 75 mg

Protein: 24 g

Sodium: 360 mg

Calcium: 35 mg

Diabetic exchanges: 3 lean meat

White Bean Cassoulet
Yield: 5 servings

2 tablespoons extra virgin olive oil

3 cups sliced fresh mushrooms

2 medium yellow onions, thinly sliced and cut into quarter rings (1 1/2 cups)

2 carrots, halved lengthwise and thinly sliced (1 cup)

3/4 cup thinly sliced celery

2 teaspoons crushed garlic

2 teaspoons dried sage

1 teaspoon whole fennel seeds

1 teaspoon dried thyme

1/2 teaspoon ground black pepper

2 cups chopped fresh plum tomatoes

1 cup V-8 juice

2 cans (15-ounces each) cannellini or white beans, drained

TOPPING
1 slice whole grain bread, torn into pieces

2 teaspoon crushed garlic

2 teaspoons extra virgin olive oil

Preheat the oven to 350 degrees F. Place the olive oil in a large nonstick skillet and add the next 9 ingredients (mushrooms through pepper). Cover and cook over medium heat for 10 minutes, stirring occasionally, until the vegetables are tender. Add the tomatoes and V-8 juice; cover and cook for about 5 minutes more, or until the tomatoes have cooked down into a thick sauce. Stir in the beans and cook for another minute to heat through. Set aside.

To make the topping, place the bread, garlic, and olive oil in a food processor and process into crumbs. Set aside. Coat five 12-ounce ramekins with cooking spray and divide the bean mixture among the ramekins. Top the bean mixture in each ramekin with some of the crumbs.

Bake uncovered for about 15 minutes, until the crumbs are lightly toasted. Let sit for 5 minutes before serving. (Alternatively, bake in a 2-quart casserole dish for about 20 minutes.)

Nutritional Facts (per 1 1/2-cup serving):
Calories: 281
Carbohydrates: 42 g
Fiber: 10.7 g
Fat: 8.7 g
Sat fat: 1.1 g
Cholesterol: 0 mg
Protein: 10.4 g
Sodium: 549 mg
Calcium: 100 mg
Diabetic exchanges: 1 1/2 lean meat, 1 1/2 starch, 2 vegetable, 1 fat

Roasted Ratatouille
Yield: 4 servings

1 pound plum tomatoes, sliced lengthwise into 3/4-inch wedges
2 cups diced peeled eggplant (3/4-inch cubes)
2 medium-small zucchini, halved lengthwise and sliced 3/4-inch thick (2 cups)

2 medium yellow onions, cut into 3/4-inch wedges
3/4 cup green bell pepper (3/4-inch pieces)
3/4 cup red bell pepper (3/4-inch pieces)
6 cloves garlic, cut into thin slivers
1 teaspoon dried thyme
1/2 teaspoon sea salt
1/2 teaspoon ground black pepper
Olive oil cooking spray
1 tablespoon extra virgin olive oil
2 cups cooked brown rice or whole wheat couscous
3 to 4 tablespoons finely chopped fresh parsley
1/2 cup shredded reduced-fat mozzarella cheese

Preheat the oven to 450 degrees F. Coat an 11-by-14-inch roasting pan with cooking spray and add the vegetables and garlic. Sprinkle with the thyme, salt, and pepper, and toss to mix. Spray the top of the vegetable mixture lightly with the cooking spray.

Bake uncovered for about 25 to 35 minutes, stirring after 10 minutes and then every 5 to 8 minutes thereafter. Cook until the vegetables are tender and browned in spots. Toss in the olive oil. Serve hot over the rice or couscous, topping each serving with some of the parsley and cheese.

Nutritional Facts (per serving):
Calories: 263
Carbohydrates: 43 g
Fiber: 7.3 g
Fat: 7.3 g
Sat fat: 2.2 g
Cholesterol: 8 mg
Protein: 9.6 g
Sodium: 377 mg
Calcium: 152 mg
Diabetic exchanges: 1/2 medium-fat meat, 1 1/2 starch, 3 vegetable, 1 fat

Chapter 16
AGE-Less Side Dishes

Choosing smart side dishes is pivotal to the AGE-Less Way. Fortunately, this is easily accomplished since vegetables, fruits, and whole grains are naturally low in AGEs. As a bonus, these super nutritious plant foods supply a bounty of inflammation-fighting phytonutrients. On the other hand, side dishes take a turn for the worse if they are deep-fried (as in French fries) or if they are drenched with butter, oil, cheese, or other fatty ingredients, which can add unhealthy amounts of AGEs.

Have a taste for grilled, broiled, or roasted foods? Sides are a great way to satisfy this craving, since grilled, broiled, or roasted vegetables will contain far fewer AGEs than meats prepared in this manner. If you want to keep meals simple, you will be happy to know that the two magic meal words—fast and easy—are also applicable here. This chapter offers a selection of easy and delicious side dishes to round out your AGE-Less meals.

Broiled Asparagus & Onions
Yield: 4 servings

1 pound fresh asparagus spears
1 large yellow onion or 1 medium-small red onion, sliced and cut into half rings
1/4 teaspoon sea salt
Scant 1/4 teaspoon ground black pepper
Olive oil cooking spray

Rinse the asparagus with cool water, shake off the excess water, and snap off the tough ends. Coat an 11-by-17-inch rimmed baking sheet with cooking spray and place the asparagus on the sheet. Top with the onions. Sprinkle with the salt and pepper and spray lightly with the cooking spray. Broil under a preheated broiler for about 10 minutes, shaking the pan every 3 minutes, until tender and nicely browned. Serve hot.

Nutritional Facts (per serving):
Calories: 35
Carbohydrates: 7 g
Fiber: 2.5 g
Fat: 0.3 g
Sat. Fat: 0.1 g
Cholesterol: 0 mg
Protein: 2.4 g
Sodium: 147 mg
Calcium: 26 mg
Diabetic exchanges: 1 vegetable

Smashed Potatoes with Garlic & Chives
Yield: 5 servings

3 1/2 cups 1-inch chunks unpeeled red-skinned new potatoes or Yukon gold potatoes, scrubbed (about 18 ounces)
4 to 6 cloves fresh garlic
1/2 cup nonfat or light sour cream
Scant 1/2 teaspoon sea salt
Scant 1/4 teaspoon ground black pepper
1 1/2 tablespoons finely chopped fresh chives

Place the potatoes and garlic in a 2-quart pot and add enough water to just cover the potatoes. Bring to a boil, then reduce the heat to medium; cover and cook for about 12 minutes or until tender. Drain and place 1/4 cup of the cooking liquid aside as a reserve.

Pick out the garlic cloves and mash with a fork; add back to the potatoes. Add the sour cream, salt, and pepper, and stir to mix. Mash the potatoes with a potato masher just enough to make them creamy but still with good sized chunks of potatoes. Stir in the chives. Add some of the reserved cooking water if the mixture seems too stiff. Serve hot.

Nutritional Facts (per 1/2-cup serving):
Calories: 89
Carbohydrates: 20 g
Fiber: 2.1 g
Fat: 0.2 g
Sat. Fat: 0 g
Cholesterol: 0 mg
Protein: 3.7 g
Sodium: 216 mg
Calcium: 51 mg
Diabetic exchanges: 1 starch

Spicy Oven Fries
Yield: 4 servings

1 1/4 pounds unpeeled Yukon Gold potatoes, scrubbed and patted dry (about 4 medium)
1 teaspoon ground paprika
1 teaspoon Cajun or Greek seasoning
Olive oil cooking spray

Preheat the oven to 400 degrees F. Cut the potatoes into strips that are about 3/8-inch thick and place in a large bowl. Add the paprika and the Cajun or Greek seasoning and toss to mix.

Coat 2 large baking sheets with cooking spray and arrange the potatoes in a single layer (not touching) on the sheets. Spray the potatoes lightly with the cooking spray and bake for 10 minutes. Turn the potatoes and bake for an additional 10 minutes or until tender and nicely browned. Serve immediately.

Nutritional Facts (per serving):

Calories: 98

Carbohydrates: 25 g

Fiber: 3 g

Fat: 0.4 g

Sat. Fat: 0.1 g

Cholesterol: 0 mg

Protein: 3.9 g

Sodium: 118 mg

Calcium: 20 mg

Diabetic exchanges: 1 1/2 starch

Vegetable Fried Rice
Yield: 5 servings

4 cups fresh or frozen (unthawed) stir-fry vegetable medley (such as broccoli, snow peas, mushrooms, and red bell peppers)
1 tablespoon canola oil
2 teaspoons finely grated fresh ginger
2 tablespoons reduced-sodium soy sauce
3 cups cooked brown rice
2 tablespoons non-toasted sesame seeds

Coat a large deep nonstick skillet with cooking spray and add the vegetables and 2 tablespoons of water or broth. Cover and cook over medium heat for about 5 minutes, shaking the pan occasionally, until the vegetables are heated through and crisp-tender. Add a little more water or broth during cooking if necessary, but only enough to prevent scorching. Add the canola oil, ginger, and soy sauce and stir to mix. Add the rice and toss for a minute or two to heat through. Toss in the sesame seeds and serve hot.

Nutritional Facts (per 1-cup serving):

Calories: 193

Carbohydrates: 32 g

Fiber: 3.7 g

Fat: 5.3 g

Sat. Fat: 0.4 g

Cholesterol: 0 mg

Protein: 6.8 g

Sodium: 201 mg

Calcium: 20 mg

Diabetic exchanges: 1 1/2 starch, 1 vegetable, 1 fat

Fried Rice with Spinach & Sesame
Yield: 5 servings

1 tablespoon canola oil
1/2 cup thin matchstick strips carrots
1/2 cup sliced scallions
2 teaspoons crushed garlic
8 cups (moderately packed) fresh spinach, chopped
2 tablespoons reduced-sodium soy sauce
2 tablespoons orange juice
2 teaspoons finely grated fresh ginger
1/4 teaspoon ground black pepper
3 cups cooked brown rice
2 tablespoons non-toasted sesame seeds

Pour the oil into a large deep nonstick skillet and add the carrots, scallions, and 1 tablespoon of water. Cover and cook over medium heat for about 4 minutes, shaking the pan occasionally, until the vegetables soften. Add a little more water during cooking if needed. Add the garlic and cook for another 15 seconds.

Add the spinach, soy sauce, orange juice, ginger, and pepper and toss to mix. Cover and cook for a couple of minutes or until the spinach wilts. Add the rice and cook uncovered for a couple of minutes to heat through and evaporate any excess liquid. Toss in the sesame seeds and serve hot.

Nutritional Facts (per 7/8-cup serving):

Calories: 183

Carbohydrates: 32 g

Fiber: 3.9 g

Fat: 4.4 g

Sat. Fat: 0.3 g

Cholesterol: 0 mg

Protein: 6.8 g

Sodium: 296 mg

Calcium: 82 mg

Diabetic exchanges: 1 1/2 starch, 1 vegetable, 1 fat

Cauliflower & Couscous Pilaf
Yield: 4 servings

1 tablespoon olive oil
1/2 cup chopped yellow onion
3 cups small fresh cauliflower florets (1/4 to 1/2-inch pieces)
3/4 cup vegetable or chicken broth
1/4 cup orange juice
1/4 cup golden raisins
2/3 cup whole wheat couscous
1/4 teaspoon sea salt
1/8 teaspoon ground white pepper
1/4 cup finely chopped fresh parsley

Pour the olive oil into a large nonstick skillet and add the onion, cauliflower, and 1/4 cup of water. Cover and cook over medium heat for about 8 minutes or until tender. Add a little more water during cooking if needed to prevent scorching.

Add the remaining ingredients except for the parsley; cover and bring to a boil. Reduce the heat and simmer for 2 minutes or until the liquid is absorbed. Sprinkle the parsley over the top and place the lid back on. Remove from the heat and let sit for 5 minutes. Fluff with a fork to mix in the parsley, and serve hot.

Nutritional Facts (per 1-cup serving):
Calories: 170
Carbohydrates: 31 g
Fiber: 4.9 g
Fat: 4.1 g
Sat. Fat: 0.5 g
Cholesterol: 0 mg
Protein: 5.9 g
Sodium: 328 mg
Calcium: 37 mg
Diabetic exchanges: 1 1/2 starch, 1 vegetable, 1 fat

Greek Broccoli Salad
Yield: 8 servings

3 cups chopped fresh broccoli florets (about 1/4-inch dice)
1 1/2 cups canned garbanzo beans, drained
1 1/2 cups chopped plum tomatoes
3/4 cup chopped red onion
1/2 cup plus 1 tablespoon light olive oil vinaigrette salad dressing
1/4 cup crumbled reduced-fat feta cheese (optional)

Combine the broccoli, garbanzo beans, tomatoes, and onion in a large bowl. Pour the dressing over the salad and toss to mix. Cover and chill for several hours or overnight before serving. If desired, toss in the feta cheese just before serving.

Nutritional Facts (per 3/4-cup serving):
Calories: 90
Carbohydrates: 11 g
Fiber: 3 g
Fat: 4.1 g
Sat. Fat: 0.3 g
Cholesterol: 0 mg
Protein: 3.3 g

Sodium: 227 mg
Calcium: 29 mg
Diabetic exchanges: 1 vegetable, 1/2 starch, 1 fat

Colorful Chopped Salad
Yield: 4 servings

6 cups thinly sliced romaine lettuce
3/4 cup chopped cauliflower
3/4 cup chopped broccoli florets
1/3 cup shredded carrot
1/2 cup sliced scallions
1/2 cup shredded reduced-fat mozzarella or cheddar cheese
1/4 cup dried cranberries
1/4 cup chopped pecans or walnuts
1/2 cup nonfat or light balsamic or olive oil vinaigrette salad dressing

Combine all of the ingredients except for the dressing in a large bowl. Drizzle the dressing over the salad and toss to mix. Serve immediately.

Nutritional Facts (per serving):
Calories: 147
Carbohydrates: 14 g
Cholesterol: 8 mg
Fat: 8.2 g
Sat. Fat: 2 g
Fiber: 4 g
Protein: 7 g
Sodium: 346 mg
Calcium: 162 mg
Diabetic exchanges: 1 carbohydrate, ½ medium-fat meat, 1 fat

Greek Chopped Salad
Yield: 6 servings

1 1/2 cups diced peeled and seeded cucumber
1 1/2 cups chopped fresh tomato
1/2 medium red onion, cut into thin wedges (1 cup)
1/2 cup finely chopped fresh parsley
3 to 4 tablespoons chopped Kalamata olives

DRESSING
1 tablespoon lemon juice
1 tablespoon red wine vinegar
1 1/2 tablespoons extra virgin olive oil
1/2 teaspoon sea salt
1/2 teaspoon ground black pepper

Combine the cucumber, tomato, onion, parsley and olives in a medium bowl.

Combine the dressing ingredients in a small bowl and stir to mix. Pour the dressing over the salad and toss to mix. Cover and chill for at least 30 minutes before serving.

Nutritional Facts (per 2/3-cup serving):
Calories: 61
Carbohydrates: 6 g
Fiber: 1.6 g
Fat: 4.1 g
Sat. Fat: 0.6 g
Cholesterol: 0 mg
Protein: 1 g
Sodium: 235 mg
Calcium: 23 mg
Diabetic exchanges: 1 vegetable, 1 fat

Garden Fresh Tabbouleh

Yield: 8 servings

1 cup uncooked bulgur wheat
1 1/2 cups chopped fresh tomatoes
1 1/2 cups chopped peeled and seeded cucumber
1 cup (packed) finely chopped fresh parsley
3/4 cup sliced scallions
1/3 cup finely chopped fresh mint

DRESSING
2 to 3 tablespoons extra virgin olive oil
3 tablespoons lemon juice
1/2 teaspoon sea salt
1/2 teaspoon ground black pepper

Prepare the bulgur wheat according to package directions and let cool.

Place the bulgur wheat, tomatoes, cucumber, parsley, scallions, and mint in a large bowl. Combine the dressing ingredients in a small bowl and stir to mix. Pour the dressing over the salad and toss to mix. Cover and chill for at least 1 hour before serving.

Nutritional Facts (per 7/8-cup serving):
Calories: 120
Carbohydrates: 17 g
Fiber: 4.4 g
Fat: 5.5 g
Sat. Fat: 0.8 g
Cholesterol: 0 mg
Protein: 3.1 g
Sodium: 157 mg
Calcium: 36 mg
Diabetic exchanges: 1 starch, 1 vegetable, 1 fat

Barley Salad with Broccoli, Corn, & Tomatoes
Yield: 8 servings

1 cup uncooked pearl barley
2 cups finely chopped fresh broccoli florets
1 cup frozen whole kernel corn, thawed
1 cup chopped plum tomatoes
3/4 cup sliced scallions
1/2 cup finely chopped fresh parsley

DRESSING
2 1/2 tablespoons extra virgin olive oil
2 1/2 tablespoons white wine vinegar
1 teaspoon crushed garlic
3/4 teaspoon sea salt
1/2 teaspoon ground black pepper

Cook the barley according to package directions. Let cool. Place the barley, broccoli, corn, tomatoes, scallions, and parsley in a large bowl and toss to mix. Combine the dressing ingredients in a small bowl, and whisk to mix. Pour the dressing over the salad and toss to mix. Cover and chill for at least 1 hour before serving.

Nutritional Facts (per 7/8-cup serving):
Calories: 141
Carbohydrates: 24 g
Fiber: 4 g
Fat: 4.8 g
Sat. Fat: 0.7 g
Cholesterol: 0 mg
Protein: 3 g
Sodium: 227 mg
Calcium: 26 mg
Diabetic exchanges: 1 starch, 1 vegetable, 1 fat

Citrus-Avocado Salad
Yield: 4 servings

8 cups chopped romaine lettuce
4 thin slices red or sweet white onion, cut into quarter-rings
1 cup fresh orange or grapefruit sections, well drained
1 cup diced avocado
1/2 cup shredded reduced-fat Monterey Jack cheese
1/4 cup plus 2 tablespoons light olive oil vinaigrette salad dressing
Freshly ground black pepper

Combine all of the ingredients except for the dressing and pepper in a large bowl. Add the dressing, sprinkle with some black pepper, and toss to mix. Serve immediately.

Nutritional Facts (per serving):
Calories: 186
Carbohydrates: 15 g
Fiber: 5.3 g
Fat: 12.8 g
Sat. fat: 2.8 g
Cholesterol: 7 mg
Protein: 7.4 g
Sodium: 280 mg
Calcium: 168 mg
Diabetic exchanges: 1/2 fruit, 2 vegetable, 2 fat

Cucumber & Tomato Salad
Yield: 6 servings

1 medium-large hothouse cucumber
4 slices red onion, cut into quarter-rings
2 tablespoons red wine vinegar
1 teaspoon sugar
Scant 1/2 teaspoon sea salt
1/4 teaspoon ground black pepper

2 cups diced plum tomato
3 to 4 tablespoons finely chopped fresh basil or parsley
1 tablespoon extra virgin olive oil

Cut the cucumber in half lengthwise and use a melon baller or spoon to scrape out the seeds. Cut the halves into 1/4-inch thick slices (there should be about 2 cups). Place in a bowl and add the onion, vinegar, sugar, salt, and pepper and toss to mix. Cover and chill for at least 1 hour. About 30 minutes before serving, stir in the tomatoes, basil, and olive oil.

Nutritional Facts (per 2/3-cup serving):
Calories: 50
Carbohydrates: 7 g
Fiber: 1.5 g
Fat: 2.5 g
Sat. Fat: 0.4 g
Cholesterol: 0 mg
Protein: 1.1 g
Sodium: 173 mg
Calcium: 15 mg
Diabetic exchanges: 1 1/2 vegetable, 1/2 fat

Green Bean & Grape Tomato Salad
Yield: 6 servings

5 cups 1-inch pieces fresh or frozen green beans
1 cup grape tomatoes, halved
2/3 cup sweet white or red onion, thinly sliced and cut into quarter-rings
2 tablespoons finely chopped fresh basil (or 2 teaspoons dried) or 1 table-
spoon finely chopped fresh dill (or 1 teaspoon dried)

DRESSING
2 tablespoons white wine vinegar
2 tablespoons extra virgin olive oil
2 teaspoons honey or sugar

1 teaspoon Dijon mustard
1/2 teaspoon sea salt
1/2 teaspoon ground black pepper

Bring a large pot of water to a boil and add the green beans. Cook and cover for about 4 minutes or until the beans are tender. You could also steam instead for about 7 minutes, until tender. Drain, rinse with cold water, and drain again.

Place the beans in a large bowl and add the tomatoes, onion, and basil. Combine all of the dressing ingredients in a small bowl and whisk to mix. Pour the dressing over the salad and toss to mix. Cover and chill for several hours or overnight before serving.

Nutritional Facts (per 3/4-cup serving):
Calories: 86
Carbohydrates: 11 g
Fiber: 2.8 g
Fat: 4.8 g
Sat. Fat: 0.7 g
Cholesterol: 0 mg
Protein: 1.8 g
Sodium: 215 mg
Calcium: 39 mg
Diabetic exchanges: 1 1/2 vegetable, 1 fat

Southwestern Cabbage Salad
Yield: 6 servings

5 cups shredded coleslaw mix or thinly sliced green cabbage
1 cup fresh cooked or frozen (thawed) whole kernel corn
1/2 cup thinly sliced scallions
1/4 cup plus 2 tablespoons chopped red bell pepper
2 to 3 tablespoons finely chopped fresh cilantro

DRESSING
2 tablespoons extra virgin olive oil
3 tablespoons white wine vinegar
1 1/2 tablespoons honey
1 teaspoon Dijon mustard
1/2 teaspoon ground cumin
Scant 1/2 teaspoon sea salt
Scant 1/2 teaspoon ground black pepper

Combine the coleslaw mix or cabbage, corn, scallions, bell pepper, and cilantro in a large bowl. Combine the dressing ingredients and whisk to mix. Pour the dressing over the salad and toss to mix. Cover and chill for several hours or overnight before serving.

Nutritional Facts (per 3/4-cup serving):
Calories: 106
Carbohydrates: 16 g
Fiber: 2.7 g
Fat: 5 g
Sat. fat: 0.7 g
Cholesterol: 0 mg
Protein: 2.1 g
Sodium: 191 mg
Calcium: 39
Diabetic exchanges: 1 carbohydrate, 1 fat

Asian Slaw with Almonds
Yield: 7 servings

6 cups thinly sliced Napa or green cabbage
3/4 cup sliced scallions
1/2 cup finely chopped fresh cilantro
1/2 cup grated carrots

3/4 cup frozen green peas
1/3 cup sliced almonds

DRESSING
1/4 cup rice vinegar
2 tablespoons canola oil
2 tablespoons honey
1 tablespoon reduced-sodium soy sauce
2 teaspoons finely grated fresh ginger
1/2 teaspoon ground black pepper
Scant 1/2 teaspoon sea salt

Combine the cabbage, scallions, cilantro, carrots, peas, and almonds in a large bowl. Combine the dressing ingredients in a small bowl and whisk to mix. Pour the dressing over the salad and toss to mix. Cover and chill for 8 hours or overnight before serving.

Nutritional Facts (per 3/4-cup serving):
Calories: 113
Carbohydrates: 13 g
Fiber: 3.6 g
Fat: 6.5 g
Sat. Fat: 0.5 g
Cholesterol: 0 mg
Protein: 3.2 g
Sodium: 123 mg
Calcium: 65 mg
Diabetic exchanges: 1 carbohydrate, 1 fat

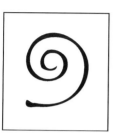

Chapter 17
Sauces and Salsas:
AGE-Less and Taste-Full

A common statement we hear is that cooking with less heat and more water is eminently tasteless. This is far from the fact. One thing to consider is that our taste for food is culturally ingrained, and new tastes can be learned even after living for many years in a particular environment. Almost every culture has its own creation of colorful, tasty and spicy sauces or salsas that significantly enhance the taste of meats, poultry, and seafood. These sauces and salsas add a strong bite, which can jazz up the flavor of an otherwise mild dish. This chapter provides a few such recipes, understanding there are many other ones you can use. Serve with poached or steamed fish or chicken, stewed beef, lamb, or pork, or even toss with vegetables, pasta, or rice for a vibrant taste sensation in AGE-Less style.

Mexican Salsa Verde
Yield: about 2 cups

1 lb fresh tomatillos
1/3 cup chopped white onion
1 to 3 tablespoons seeded and chopped jalapeño pepper
1/3 cup chopped fresh cilantro leaves
2 teaspoons fresh lime juice
1/2 teaspoon sea salt
Scant 1/4 teaspoon sugar

Remove the papery husks from the tomatillos and rinse well. Place the tomatillos in a saucepan and cover with water. Bring to a boil and cook for 5 minutes or until softened. Remove the tomatillos with a slotted spoon and transfer to a blender.

Add the remaining ingredients to the blender and blend until the ingredients are finely chopped and mixed. Cool in the refrigerator. Serve as an accompaniment to Mexican dishes or with baked tortilla chips.

Nutritional Facts (per 1/4-cup serving)
Calories: 22
Carbohydrates: 4 g
Fiber: 1.3 g
Fat: 0.6 g
Sat. Fat: 0.1 g
Cholesterol: 0 mg
Protein: 0.7 g
Sodium: 145 mg
Calcium: 7 mg
Diabetic exchanges: free food

Chilean Pebre (Cilantro Sauce)
Yield: about 2 cups

1 medium tomato, chopped
1 small onion, chopped
2 medium mild chili peppers (such as banana peppers), seeded and chopped
1 clove garlic, crushed
2 cups fresh cilantro leaves, finely chopped
1 tablespoon lemon juice
1 tablespoon red wine vinegar
2 tablespoons extra virgin olive oil
1/2 teaspoon sea salt
1/4 teaspoon ground black pepper

Combine all of the ingredients and stir to mix. Serve with fish, poultry, or meat. This sauce is best freshly made but can be refrigerated for several hours before serving. If chilled, return to room temperature before serving.

Nutritional Facts (per 1/4-cup serving)
Calories: 43
Carbohydrates: 1 g
Fiber: 1.1 g
Fat: 3.5 g
Sat. Fat: 0.5 g
Cholesterol: 0 mg
Protein: 0.7 g
Sodium: 153 mg
Calcium: 12 mg
Diabetic exchanges: 1/2 fat

Lemon-Parsley Sauce
Yield: about 7/8 cup

1 teaspoon crushed garlic
1/2 teaspoon sea salt
1/4 teaspoon ground black pepper
1/4 teaspoon dried crushed red pepper
1/2 teaspoon freshly grated lemon rind
1/4 cup lemon juice
1 tablespoon water
1/4 cup plus 2 tablespoons extra-virgin olive oil
1/2 cup (packed) fresh parsley leaves, finely chopped
1 tablespoons capers, drained

Mix the first 5 ingredients in small bowl and mash into a paste. Whisk in the lemon juice and water. Add the olive oil in thin stream, whisking constantly, until blended. Stir in the parsley and capers. If desired, season with more pepper. Let stand for 20 minutes before serving, or cover and chill for up to several hours before serving. If chilled, return to room temperature and stir well before using. Spoon a small amount over a portion of fish, poultry, or meat.

Nutritional Facts (per tablespoon)
Calories: 54
Carbohydrates: 1 g
Fiber: 0.1 g
Fat: 5.8 g
Sat. Fat: 0.8 g
Cholesterol: 0 mg
Protein: 0.1 g
Sodium: 101 mg
Calcium: 4 mg
Diabetic exchanges: 1 fat

Chimichurri Sauce
Yield: about 3/4 cup

1/2 cup (packed) fresh parsley leaves, finely chopped
1 tablespoon fresh oregano, finely chopped (or 1 teaspoon dried oregano)
1/4 cup extra virgin olive oil
1/4 cup lemon juice, white wine vinegar, or red wine vinegar
1 tablespoon water
1 teaspoon crushed garlic
1/2 teaspoon sea salt
1/4teaspoon freshly ground black pepper
1/4 teaspoon dried red pepper flakes

Place the parsley and oregano in a small bowl. Stir in the remaining ingredients. If desired, season with more pepper. Let stand for 20 minutes before serving, or refrigerate for up to 2 days. If chilled, return to room temperature and stir well before serving. Spoon a small amount over a portion of fish, poultry, or meat.

Nutritional Facts (per tablespoon)

Calories: 42

Carbohydrates: 1 g

Fiber: 0.1 g

Fat: 4.5 g

Sat. Fat: 0.6 g

Cholesterol: 0 mg

Protein: 0.2 g

Sodium: 97 mg

Calcium: 6 mg

Diabetic exchanges: 1 fat

Basil Pesto
Yield: about 1 1/2 cups

2 cups (packed) fresh basil leaves
1/4 cup grated Parmesan cheese
1/2 cup extra virgin olive oil
3 tablespoons walnuts
3 garlic cloves, finely minced
1/4 teaspoon sea salt

Combine all of the ingredients in a food processor. Process until smooth, stopping periodically to scrape down the sides. Toss a small amount with pasta, rice, or steamed vegetables, or spread over a portion of steamed fish. Basil pesto can be kept in refrigerator for up to one week, or freeze for a few months.

Nutritional Facts (per tablespoon)

Calories: 53

Carbohydrates: 0.3 g

Fiber: 0.2 g

Fat: 5.6 g

Sat. Fat: 0.9 g

Cholesterol: 1 mg
Protein: 0.8 g
Sodium: 43 mg
Calcium: 20 mg
Diabetic exchanges: 1 fat

⊙ Chapter 18
Smart Snacks

Smart snacking is key to success on the AGE-Less Way. The solution is simple: snack on "real food" instead of the chips, crackers, cookies, creamy-sugary coffee drinks, and other grab-and-go fare that we are conditioned to think of as snacks. As you know by now, processed snacks are often heat-treated, high in fat and/or sugar, and disproportionately high in AGEs. There are many convenient but lower-AGE choices such as fruit, yogurt, or a low-fat latte with a sprinkling of cocoa. A cup of soup, a small bowl of cereal, or leftovers from an AGE-Less meal is also a good choice for lower-AGE snacks. Again, think "real food." This chapter features some additional recipes that can fit the bill for smart snacking.

Creamy Artichoke Spread
Yield: about 1 1/4 cups

15-ounce can artichoke hearts, well drained
1/4 cup plus 2 tablespoons nonfat or low-fat mayonnaise
2 tablespoons light garlic & herb-flavored cream cheese

Chop the artichokes and place in wire strainer. Press to remove as much of the liquid as possible. Place the drained artichokes in the bowl of a food processor and add the mayonnaise and cream cheese. Process until the artichokes are finely chopped and the mixture is creamy. Add a little more mayonnaise if desired.

Serve immediately or cover and refrigerate until ready to serve. Serve with carrot and celery sticks, wedges of whole grain pita bread or slices of whole grain bagels. You can also use it as a sandwich spread.

Nutritional Facts (per 1/4-cup serving):

Calories: 52

Carbohydrates: 8 g

Fiber: 2 g

Fat: 1.2 g

Sat. Fat: 0.8 g

Cholesterol: 4 mg

Protein: 2.4 g

Sodium: 240 mg

Calcium: 8 mg

Diabetic exchanges: 1/2 carbohydrate

Spicy Garbanzo Spread
Yield: about 1 1/2 cups

2/3 cup chopped red or yellow bell pepper
2/3 cup chopped yellow onion
1 to 2 tablespoons extra virgin olive oil
2 teaspoons crushed garlic
1 teaspoon ground cumin
15-ounce can chickpeas (garbanzo beans) drained
1/4 teaspoon crushed red pepper flakes
1/4 teaspoon ground black pepper
2 tablespoons plain nonfat or low-fat yogurt
2 teaspoons lemon juice
1/4 teaspoon sea salt

Coat a medium-small nonstick skillet with cooking spray and add the peppers, onion, and 2 tablespoons of water. Cover and cook over medium heat for several minutes to soften. Add the olive oil, garlic, and cumin and cook with the cover on for another 30 seconds.

Place the cooked vegetable mixture in the bowl of a food processor and add the remaining ingredients. Process until smooth, adding a little more yogurt if needed. Serve immediately or cover and chill. Serve with carrot and celery sticks and wedges of whole grain pita bread. Can also be used as a sandwich filling.

Nutritional Facts (per 1/4 cup):
Calories: 104
Carbohydrate: 15 g
Fiber: 3.8 g
Fat: 3.5 g
Sat. Fat: 0.4 g
Cholesterol: 0 mg
Protein: 4.4 g
Sodium: 201 mg
Calcium: 40 mg
Diabetic exchanges: 1 starch, 1/2 fat

Herbed White Bean Spread
Yield: about 1 1/4 cups

15-ounce can cannellini beans or white beans, rinsed and drained
1 1/2 tablespoons lemon juice
1 1/2 tablespoons extra virgin olive oil
1 1/2 teaspoons chopped fresh rosemary or 1/2 teaspoon dried
1 1/2 teaspoons chopped fresh sage or 1/2 teaspoon dried
1 teaspoon crushed garlic
1/4 teaspoon coarsely ground black pepper

Place all of the ingredients in a food processor and process until smooth. Serve immediately with fresh cut vegetables or whole grain pita wedges. You can also cover and chill, but bring to room temperature before serving.

Nutritional Facts (per 1/4 cup):
Calories: 98
Carbohydrate: 12 g

Fiber: 3.1 g
Fat: 4.4 g
Sat. Fat: 0.6 g
Cholesterol: 0 mg
Protein: 3.1 g
Sodium: 97 mg
Calcium: 28 mg
Diabetic exchanges: 1 starch, 1 fat

Roasted Eggplant Spread
Yield: about 2 cups

1 large eggplant (1 1/4 pounds), cut in half lengthwise
1 medium yellow onion, cut into 1/2-inch-thick slices
1 plum tomato, cut in half lengthwise
Olive oil cooking spray
10 fresh garlic cloves (about 1 medium head)
1/4 cup finely chopped fresh parsley or 4 teaspoons dried
1 tablespoon lemon juice
1 tablespoon extra-virgin olive oil
1/2 teaspoon sea salt
1/2 teaspoon ground black pepper

Preheat the oven to 400 degrees F. Coat a large baking sheet with cooking spray and place the eggplant halves, cut side down, on the sheet. Pierce at 1-inch intervals with a fork. Add onion slices and tomato halves (cut side up) to the baking sheet. Spray the onion and tomatoes lightly with cooking spray.

Coat an 8-inch piece of aluminum foil with cooking spray and place the garlic on the bottom half. Fold the top over and tightly seal the edges to form a packet. Place on the baking sheet with the vegetables.

Roast the vegetables and garlic for 15 minutes. Turn the onion slices over and bake for about 10 minutes more or until the onions are tender and browned. Remove the onion, tomatoes, and garlic to a cutting board and set aside.

Return the eggplant to the oven and bake for about 15 minutes more, or until very soft. Let cool slightly. Slip off and discard the eggplant skins and chop the flesh. Place the flesh in a wire strainer and set over a bowl for 30 minutes to drain.

Unwrap the garlic and place in a medium bowl. Mash with a fork. Add the drained eggplant and the tomatoes, and mash to the desired consistency. Finely chop the onion and add to the bowl. Stir in the parsley, lemon juice, oil, salt, and pepper. Serve immediately or cover and chill until ready to serve. Bring to room temperature before serving. Serve with wedges of whole grain pita bread.

Nutritional Facts (per 1/4 cup serving):
Calories: 42
Carbohydrates: 6 g
Fiber: 1.8 g
Fat: 1.9 g
Sat. fat: 0.3 g
Cholesterol: 0 mg
Protein: 1.1 g
Sodium: 148 mg
Calcium: 17 mg
Diabetic exchanges: 1 vegetable, 1/2 fat

Yogurt-Raisin-Walnut Spread
Yield: 1 1/4 cups

1 cup nonfat or low-fat yogurt cheese* or Greek-style yogurt
2 tablespoons honey
1/4 cup raisins
3 tablespoons chopped walnuts
Pinch ground cinnamon (optional)

Combine the yogurt cheese or Greek yogurt and honey in a small bowl and stir to mix. Fold in the raisins and walnuts. Cover and chill for at least 8 hours before serving. Use as a topping for bagels or serve with sliced apples or pears.

Nutritional Facts (per 1/4 cup serving):
Calories: 110
Carbohydrate: 18 g
Fiber: 0.5 g
Fat: 2.8 g
Sat. Fat: 0.2 g
Cholesterol: 1 mg
Protein: 4.9 g
Sodium: 36 mg
Calcium: 97 mg
Diabetic exchanges: 1 carbohydrate, 1/2 fat

*Yogurt cheese is a creamy, protein-rich alternative to high-AGE cream cheese (it is similar to Greek-style yogurt, but a little thicker). Use yogurt cheese on bagels or as a base for dips and spreads.

- Line a strainer with 2 or 3 layers of cheesecloth or a coffee filter (or purchase a specially made yogurt cheese funnel).
- Place the strainer or funnel over a container (to catch the liquid) and spoon in the desired amount of yogurt. Important: Use a brand of yogurt that contains no gelatin, vegetable gums, or modified food starch as thickeners (pectin is okay). Use plain yogurt or try flavors such as vanilla or lemon for a change.
- Refrigerate for 8 hours or overnight, until the yogurt is reduced by half.

Oatmeal Banana Bread
Yield: 16 slices

1 1/4 cups whole-wheat pastry flour
1/2 cup quick cooking (1-minute) oats

1/2 cup light brown sugar
2 teaspoons baking powder
Scant 1/2 teaspoon ground nutmeg
1 cup very ripe mashed banana
1/4 cup nonfat or low-fat milk
1/4 cup fat-free egg substitute or 1 egg, beaten
3 tablespoons canola oil
1 teaspoon vanilla extract

Preheat the oven to 350 degrees F. Place the flour, oats, brown sugar, baking powder, and nutmeg in a large bowl, and stir to mix well. Combine the banana, milk, egg substitute or egg, oil, and vanilla and stir to mix. Add to the flour mixture, and stir just until the dry ingredients are moistened. Set the batter aside for 10 minutes.

Stir the batter for about 5 seconds. Coat a 9-by-5-inch pan or two 3 1/2-by-7-inch pans with cooking spray and spread the batter evenly in the pan. Bake for about 40 minutes (about 25 minutes if using the small pans), or until a wooden toothpick inserted in the center of the loaf comes out clean.

Cool in the pans for 15 minutes. Then remove and place on the wire rack to cool thoroughly before slicing.

Nutritional Facts (per slice):
Calories: 110
Carbohydrates: 19 g
Fiber: 1.9 g
Fat: 3 g
Sat. Fat: 0.3 g
Cholesterol: 0 mg
Protein: 2.4 g
Sodium: 72 mg
Calcium: 47 mg
Diabetic exchanges: 1 carbohydrate, 1/2 fat

For variety:

- Substitute applesauce for the mashed banana.
- Add 1/3 to 1/2 cup raisins, dates, dried cranberries, or dried blueberries to the batter just before baking.
- Add 1/3 cup chopped walnuts or pecans to the batter just before baking.

Zucchini Spice Bread
Yield: 16 slices

1 cup whole-wheat pastry flour
1/2 cup quick-cooking (1-minute) oats
2/3 cup brown sugar
1 teaspoon baking powder
1/4 teaspoon baking soda
1/2 teaspoon cinnamon
1/4 teaspoon grated nutmeg
1/4 teaspoon ground cloves
1/4 cup fat-free egg substitute or 1 egg, beaten
3 tablespoons canola oil
1 1/4 cups grated zucchini, moderately packed
1/2 cup unsweetened applesauce
1/3 cup raisins
1/4 cup chopped walnuts

Preheat the oven to 350°F. Combine the first 8 ingredients (flour through cloves) in a large bowl and stir to mix. Set aside. Combine the egg substitute or egg, oil, zucchini, and applesauce and stir to mix. Add the egg mixture to the flour mixture and stir to mix. Set the batter aside for 10 minutes and then fold in the raisins and walnuts.

Coat an 8-by-4-inch pan or two 3 1/2-by-5 1/2-inch pans with cooking spray and spread the batter evenly in the pan. Bake for about 45 minutes (about 30 minutes if using the small pans), or just until a wooden toothpick inserted in the center of the loaf comes out clean.

Cool in the pans for 15 minutes. Then remove and place on the wire rack to cool thoroughly before slicing.

Nutritional Facts (per slice):
Calories: 121
Carbohydrates: 20 g
Fiber: 1.8 g
Fat: 4 g
Sat. Fat: 0.3 g
Cholesterol: 0 mg
Protein: 2.5 g
Sodium: 63 mg
Calcium: 31 mg
Diabetic exchanges: 1 carbohydrate, 1 fat

Cool Cappuccino Frappe
Yield: 1 serving

3/4 cup coffee, frozen into ice cubes
1/2 cup nonfat or low-fat milk
1 tablespoon plus 1 teaspoon sugar-free instant white chocolate pudding mix
Sugar substitute equal to 1 to 2 tablespoons sugar
Pinch ground cinnamon (optional)

Place all of the ingredients in a blender and blend until smooth. Pour into a 16-ounce glass and serve immediately. (This recipe works best if you have a powerful blender with an ice-crushing blade.)

Nutritional Facts (per serving):
Calories: 79
Carbohydrates: 14 g
Fiber: 0 g
Fat: 0.2 g
Sat. Fat: 0.1 g

Cholesterol: 2 mg Protein: 4.3 g
Sodium: 299 mg
Calcium: 153 mg
Diabetic exchanges: 1 carbohydrate

⟳ Chapter 19
Sweets and Treats

If you enjoy a sweet treat, then you will be happy to learn that living an AGE-Less lifestyle does not necessarily mean doing without. We can, however, be smart about our sweet indulgences. Always keep in mind that rich desserts are loaded with preformed AGEs due to the large amounts of fats and sugars they contain. Remember also, that when we follow a meat meal with a rich dessert, we create even more AGEs when the fats and sugars in the dessert mix with the meat from the main course during digestion. So how can you have your dessert and eat it too? If you have a rich dessert, enjoy just a few bites. Even better, enjoy an AGE-Less treat like one presented in this chapter. As you will see, ingredients like antioxidant-rich fruits, low-fat dairy products, and wholesome whole grains can star in a dazzling array of sweet treats that minimize AGEs while maximizing satisfaction.

Moist Mocha Fudge Cake
Yield: 12 servings

2/3 cup whole wheat pastry flour
1/4 cup oat flour
1/3 cup cocoa powder
2/3 cup sugar
Sugar substitute equal to 1/3 cup sugar
1 teaspoon baking powder
1/4 teaspoon baking soda
1/4 teaspoon ground cinnamon

1/4 teaspoon sea salt
1/2 cup black coffee (room temperature)
3 tablespoons canola oil
1/4 cup fat-free egg substitute or 1 egg, beaten
1 teaspoon vanilla extract
1 cup finely chopped peeled fresh peeled pears

Preheat the oven to 350 degrees F. Combine the flours, cocoa, sugar, sugar substitute, baking powder, baking soda, cinnamon, and salt and stir to mix well. Combine the coffee, oil, egg substitute or egg, and vanilla and stir to mix. Add the coffee mixture and the pears to the flour mixture and stir to mix. Set the batter aside for 10 minutes.

Stir the batter for about 5 seconds and spread evenly into an 8-by-8-inch pan coated with cooking spray. Bake for about 25 minutes or just until the top springs back when lightly touched and a wooden toothpick inserted in the center of the cake comes out clean or coated with a few fudgy crumbs. Let the cake cool to room temperature. If desired, sift a couple of tablespoons of powdered sugar over the top just before serving.

Nutritional Facts (per serving):
Calories: 121
Carbohydrates: 21 g
Fiber: 2.3 g
Fat: 4 g
Sat. Fat: 0.4 g
Cholesterol: 0 mg
Protein: 2.3 g
Sodium: 125 mg
Calcium: 29 mg
Diabetic exchanges: 1 1/2 carbohydrate, 1 fat

For variety: Add 1/4 cup each raisins and chopped pecans or walnuts to the batter.

Steamed Apples
Yield: 4 servings

4 apples, peeled and sliced (3 cups)
1 teaspoon honey
1/8 to 1/4 teaspoon ground cinnamon

Place the apples and 1/4 cup of water in a 2-quart pot. Cover and place over medium heat. Let the apples cook for about 5 minutes or until crisp-tender.

Remove from the heat and stir in the honey and cinnamon. Cover and let sit for 20 minutes. Add a little sugar substitute for extra sweetness if desired. Serve hot or cold, plain or with yogurt.

Nutritional Facts (per 1/2-cup serving):
Calories: 53
Carbohydrates: 14 g
Fiber: 1.7 g
Fat: 0.2 g
Sat. Fat: 0 g
Cholesterol: 0 mg
Protein: 0.1 g
Sodium: 0 mg
Calcium: 4 mg
Diabetic exchanges: 1 carbohydrate

Grilled Plums with Goat Cheese
Yield: 4 servings

4 fresh plums, halved and pitted
1 tablespoon frozen (thawed) orange juice concentrate
1 tablespoon lime juice
1/4 cup crumbled soft goat cheese

Trim a small slice from the bottom of each plum half so they will sit upright. Place the plum halves on a grill or broiler pan. Combine the juice concentrate and lime juice and brush some over each plum half. Grill or broil for about 6 minutes, turning and basting every 2 minutes, until tender and nicely browned. Place 1/2 tablespoon of cheese in the center of each plum half and serve warm.

Nutritional Facts (per serving):
Calories: 63
Carbohydrates: 11 g
Fiber: 1 g
Fat: 1.9 g
Sat. Fat: 1.1 g
Cholesterol: 5 mg
Protein: 1.9 g
Sodium: 27 mg
Calcium: 31 mg
Diabetic exchanges: 1 carbohydrate

Citrus Poached Pears
Yield: 4 servings

2 large pears (8 ounces each)
1/2 cup plus 1 tablespoon orange juice
Sugar substitute equal to 2 tablespoons sugar
1 tablespoon natural cane sugar or light brown sugar
1/2 teaspoon finely grated fresh ginger*
1 1/4 teaspoons cornstarch
1 1/2 tablespoons sliced almonds

Peel the pears, halve lengthwise, and scoop out the cores. Place the pears in a 2-quart nonstick pot just large enough to hold them in a single layer. Stir together 1/2 cup of the orange juice, and all of the sugar substitute, sugar, and ginger. Pour the juice mixture over the pears.

Cover, and bring to a boil over medium heat. Reduce the heat to maintain a simmer and cook for about 8 minutes, turning after 4 minutes, until the pears are tender. Place a pear half in each of 4 small dessert dishes.

Mix the cornstarch and remaining orange juice and stir into the juices remaining in the pot. Cook and stir for about 1 minute, until thickened and bubbly. Drizzle some of the sauce over each pear half and sprinkle with some of the almonds. Serve warm.

Nutritional Facts (per serving):
Calories: 103
Carbohydrates: 23 g
Fiber: 2.7 g
Fat: 1.6 g
Sat. Fat: 0.1 g
Cholesterol: 0 mg
Protein: 1.1 g
Sodium: 1 mg
Calcium: 20 mg
Diabetic exchanges: 1 1/2 carbohydrate, 1/2 fat

*Tip: Peel a piece of fresh ginger and freeze in a freezer bag. Grate frozen ginger as needed and return the rest to the freezer for later use.

Key Lime Panna Cotta
Yield: 6 servings

3/4 cup whole milk
2 tablespoons sugar
Sugar substitute equal to 3 tablespoons sugar
3 tablespoons key lime juice
1 1/4 teaspoons unflavored gelatin
1 1/2 cups low-fat Greek-style vanilla yogurt
1 tablespoon frozen (thawed) orange juice concentrate
1 cup sliced fresh strawberries

Place half of the milk and all of the sugar in a small pot. Cook and stir over medium heat for a minute or just until the sugar dissolves. Remove from the heat and stir in the remaining milk and the sugar substitute. Set aside.

Place the lime juice in a small bowl and sprinkle the gelatin over the top. Let sit for 5 minutes. Microwave for about 20 seconds, stirring after 10 seconds, until the gelatin dissolves (do not let the juice boil). Place the yogurt in a medium-size bowl. Whisk the gelatin mixture into the yogurt, followed by the orange juice concentrate and then the milk mixture.

Divide the panna cotta mixture between six custard cups. Cover and chill for several hours or overnight. Serve in the cups, or run a knife around the edges and invert onto dessert plates. Garnish each serving with some of the strawberries.

Nutritional Facts (per serving):
Calories: 115
Carbohydrates: 18 g
Fiber: 1 g
Fat: 2.3 g
Sat. Fat: 1.4 g
Cholesterol: 9 mg
Protein: 5.8 g
Sodium: 40 mg
Calcium: 129 mg
Diabetic exchanges: 1 carbohydrate

Lemon Tapioca Pudding
Yield: 6 servings

1/4 cup minute tapioca
1 1/2 cups low-fat milk
3 tablespoons sugar
Sugar substitute equal to 2 tablespoons sugar

1/4 cup fat-free egg substitute
1 1/4 cups light lemon yogurt

Place all of the ingredients except for the yogurt in a 2-quart pot. Stir to mix, and let sit for 5 minutes. Place over medium heat and cook, stirring constantly, until the mixture comes to a full boil. Remove from the heat and let sit for 20 minutes. Whisk in the yogurt. Divide among six 6-ounce wine glasses. Cover and chill for several hours or overnight before serving.

Nutritional Facts (per 1/2 cup serving):
Calories: 115
Carbohydrates: 21 g
Fiber: 0 g
Fat: 0.7 g
Sat. Fat: 0.4 g
Cholesterol: 2 mg
Protein: 5.6 g
Sodium: 94 mg
Calcium: 174 mg
Diabetic exchanges: 1 1/2 carbohydrate

Cherry-Berry Delight
Yield: 4 servings

4-serving size package sugar-free strawberry or cranberry gelatin
3/4 cup boiling water
3/4 cup orange or pomegranate juice
2 cups frozen mixed berries, thawed and slightly crushed (non-drained)
1/2 cup frozen pitted dark sweet cherries, halved and thawed (non-drained)

Place the gelatin in a medium heatproof bowl. Pour the boiling water over the gelatin and stir for 2 minutes to dissolve the gelatin. Stir in the juice. Add the berries and cherries, along with their juices, to the gelatin mixture and stir to mix.

Divide the gelatin mixture between four 8-ounce wine glasses. Cover and chill for several hours or overnight, until firm. Garnish with a little light whipped topping just before serving if desired.

Nutritional Facts (per serving):

Calories: 69

Carbohydrates: 15 g

Fiber: 2.5 g

Fat: 0.1 g

Sat. Fat: 0 g

Cholesterol: 0 mg

Protein: 2.2 g

Sodium: 55 mg

Calcium: 16 mg

Diabetic exchanges: 1 carbohydrate

Razzleberry Gelatin
Yield: 4 servings

12 ounces sugar-free ginger ale
2 teaspoons unflavored gelatin
2 tablespoons sugar
1 1/2 cups fresh raspberries (or use half raspberries and half blackberries)

Place 1/2 cup of the ginger ale in a 1-quart pot and sprinkle the gelatin over the top. Let sit for 2 minutes to soften the gelatin. Place over low heat, and cook, stirring frequently for a couple of minutes until the gelatin is completely dissolved. Do not boil. Remove from the heat. Add the sugar and stir until it dissolves.

Slowly pour the remaining ginger ale, a few tablespoons at a time (to minimize foaming) into the gelatin mixture. Set aside for about 10 minutes to cool to room temperature.

Divide the berries among four 8-ounce wine glasses and pour one-fourth of the ginger ale mixture into each glass. Cover and chill for several hours or until set before serving.

Nutritional Facts (per serving):
Calories: 48
Carbohydrates: 11 g
Fiber: 3.1 g
Fat: 0.2 g
Sat. Fat: 0 g
Cholesterol: 0 mg
Protein: 1.2 g
Sodium: 19 mg
Calcium: 11 mg
Diabetic exchanges: 1 carbohydrate

Dark Chocolate Mousse
Yield: 6 servings

1 1/4 cups low-fat milk
1/4 cup chopped dark chocolate
1/2 teaspoon instant coffee granules
1/4 teaspoon ground cinnamon
1 package (4-serving size) sugar-free instant chocolate pudding mix
2 cups nonfat or light whipped topping

Place about 1/3 cup of the milk and all of the chocolate, coffee, and cinnamon in a 2-quart nonstick pot. Place over medium-low heat and whisk until the chocolate is completely melted. Remove from the heat and gradually whisk in the remaining milk.

Add the pudding mix to the milk mixture and whisk for 2 minutes. Place the pudding mixture in the refrigerator for 1 hour, or until well chilled and thickened. Fold half of the whipped topping into the pudding, and then fold in the rest. Spoon the mousse into six small dessert dishes and chill for at least 2 hours before serving.

If desired, garnish with fresh raspberries or strawberry slices just before serving.

Nutritional Facts (per 1/2-cup serving):
Calories: 122
Carbohydrates: 20 g
Fiber: 0.6 g
Fat: 2.7 g
Sat. Fat: 1.6 g
Cholesterol: 4 mg
Protein: 2.8 g
Sodium: 223 mg
Calcium: 70 mg
Diabetic exchanges: 1 1/2 carbohydrate, 1/2 fat

Strawberry Mousse
Yield: 4 servings

1 tablespoon cornstarch
2 cups frozen strawberries, chopped into 1/4 to 1/2 inch pieces and thawed
(do not drain)
Sugar substitute equal to 1/4 cup sugar
1 cup nonfat or low-fat Greek-style vanilla yogurt
1 cup nonfat or light whipped topping
1 1/2 tablespoons finely chopped dark chocolate (optional)
1 1/2 tablespoons sliced almonds (optional)

Place the cornstarch and 1 tablespoon of water in a small bowl and stir to dissolve the cornstarch. Set aside. Place the berries along with their liquid in a medium nonstick skillet and bring to a boil over medium heat. Cook, mashing the berries with the back of a spoon and stirring constantly, for several minutes or until the berries are reduced to about 3/4 cup in volume.

Stir the cornstarch mixture and slowly add to the strawberry mixture, while stirring constantly. Cook for about 30 seconds, or until the berries are very thick. Remove from the heat and stir in the sugar substitute. Transfer to a medium-sized bowl; cover and chill for at least 1 hour.

Stir the yogurt into the chilled berry mixture and then gently fold in the whipped topping. Divide the mousse among 4 small wine glasses and chill for at least one hour before serving. If desired, top each serving with a sprinkling of chocolate and almonds just before serving.

Nutritional Facts (per 2/3-cup serving):
Calories: 90
Carbohydrates: 16 g
Fiber: 1.6 g
Fat: 0.8 g
Sat. Fat: 0.2 g
Cholesterol: 0 mg
Protein: 6.2 g
Sodium: 30 mg
Calcium: 83 mg
Diabetic exchanges: 1 carbohydrate

Strawberry Gelato
Yield: 1 serving

1 cup coarsely chopped frozen strawberries (or use half blueberries and half strawberries)
Sugar substitute equal to 1 to 2 tablespoons sugar
1/3 cup nonfat or low-fat Greek-style vanilla yogurt

Place the berries and sugar substitute in a mini food processor and process for a minute or two, or until finely ground. Add the yogurt and process for an additional minute, scraping down the sides as needed, until smooth. Add a little more yogurt if needed. Spoon into an 8-ounce wine glass and serve immediately.

Nutritional Facts (per serving):
Calories: 106
Carbohydrates: 18 g
Fiber: 3.8 g
Fat: 0.6 g
Sat. Fat: 0 g
Cholesterol: 0 mg
Protein: 8.6 g
Sodium: 32 mg
Calcium: 117 mg
Diabetic exchanges: 1 carbohydrate

Cherry Gelato
Yield: 1 serving

3/4 cup frozen dark sweet pitted cherries
Sugar substitute equal to 1 1/2 tablespoons sugar
1/4 cup nonfat or low-fat Greek-style yogurt
2 teaspoons sliced almonds or chopped walnuts
2 teaspoons chopped dark chocolate

Place the cherries and sugar substitute in a mini food processor and process for a minute or two, or until finely ground. Add the yogurt and process for another minute, scraping down the sides as needed, until smooth. Add a little more yogurt if needed. Add the nuts and chocolate stir to mix in. Spoon into an 8-ounce wine glass and serve immediately.

Nutritional Facts (per serving)
Calories: 150
Carbohydrates: 24 g
Fiber: 3.1 g
Fat: 4.1 g
Sat. Fat: 1.4 g

Cholesterol: 0 mg

Protein: 6.2 g

Sodium: 19 mg

Calcium: 60 mg

Diabetic exchanges: 1 1/2 carbohydrate, 1 fat

Cappuccino Granita
Yield: 4 servings

1/2 cup hot coffee (use plain coffee or try hazelnut, vanilla, or other flavored coffees)
3 tablespoons natural cane sugar or light brown sugar
Sugar substitute equal to 1/4 cup sugar
1/2 cup whole milk

Place the coffee, sugar, and sugar substitute in a bowl and stir to dissolve the sugar. Let cool to room temperature. Stir in the milk. Place in a 9-by-5-inch loaf pan and freeze for 45 minutes or until partially frozen and icy around the edges.

Using a fork, scrape the frozen crystals into light shavings and stir back into the center portion. Press out any lumps with the fork. Repeat the scraping process every 45 minutes for about 2 1/2 to 3 hours or until the mixture is icy and granular. Spoon into chilled dessert dishes or wine glasses and serve.

Tip: Make the granita the day before and cover the pan with foil until ready to serve. Scrape the granita to loosen the crystals just before serving.

Nutritional Facts (per serving)

Calories: 56

Carbohydrates: 11 g

Fiber: 0 g

Fat: 1 g

Sat. Fat: 0.6 g

Cholesterol: 4 mg

Protein: 1 g

Sodium: 16 mg

Calcium: 37 mg

Diabetic exchanges: 1 carbohydrate

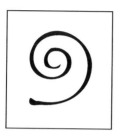

Chapter 20
AGE-Less Meal Strategies and Sample Menus

The primary goal of this book is to enable you to create your own meal plans using AGE-Less ingredients, cooking methods, and food combinations. This chapter will help you put these principles into practice. We begin by providing some simple tips for giving your diet an AGE-Less makeover. In the next section you will find six weeks of easy and delicious menus that can be enjoyed by the entire family. With a little practice, you will soon find that it is easy to turn old habits into new, healthy AGE-Less habits.

The AGE-Less Makeover

The keys to success on the AGE-Less Way are (1) to find new lower-AGE ways to prepare the foods you love, (2) to use smart substitutions for high-AGE foods, and (3) to keep portions in perspective. The following table estimates the AGE content of two daily menus featuring similar foods prepared in different ways. Note the dramatic difference that simple changes can make! AGEs are measured in kilo units, or kU. Aim for 5,000 to 8,000 kU per day.

High-AGE Menu	AGE (kU)	Low-AGE Menu	AGE (kU)
Breakfast		**Breakfast**	
Fresh fruit cup	35	Fresh fruit cup	35
Fried egg	1,200	Scrambled egg, cooking spray	30
Toasted bagel (2 oz.)	100	Untoasted bagel (2 oz.)	70
Cream cheese (2 Tbsp)	2,940	Yogurt cheese (2 Tbsp)	5
Nonfat milk (1 cup)	5	Nonfat milk (1 cup)	5
Coffee (1 cup) with	5	Coffee (1 cup) with	5
Half & half (1 Tbsp)	330	Whole milk (1/4 cup)	3
Lunch		**Lunch**	
Grilled chicken salad:		Poached chicken salad:	
Grilled chicken breast (3 oz.)	4,300	Poached chicken (3 oz.)	940
Salad greens & vegetables (3 cups)	50	Salad greens & vegetables (3 cups)	50
Shredded cheddar cheese (1/4 cup)	1,660	Light shredded cheddar cheese (1/4 cup)	740
Italian dressing (3 Tbsp)	320	Light Italian dressing (3 Tbsp)	160
Toasted wheat crackers (1 oz.)	275	Whole grain pita wedges (1 oz.)	15
Iced tea (8 oz)	5	Iced tea (8 oz)	5
Snack		**Snack**	
Apple	15	Apple	15
Processed American cheese (3/4 oz.)	1,950	Light vanilla yogurt (6 oz)	7
		Walnuts (1 Tbsp)	300
Dinner		**Dinner**	
Grilled steak (3 oz.)	6,600	Beef stew (3 oz.) over	2,200
Baked oven fries (3 oz.)	490	Mashed potatoes, low-fat recipe (3 oz.)	25
Steamed green beans (3/4 cup) with	20	Steamed green beans (3/4 cup) with	20
margarine (1 tsp)	180	untoasted sliced almonds (1 Tbsp)	300
Melon wedge	20	Melon wedge	20
TOTALS	20,500		4,950

Losing Weight the AGE-Less Way

A benefit of the AGE-Less Way is a gradual but significant weight loss without counting calories (see Chapter 2). The scientific reason for this benefit is still being refined, but it is clear that the AGE-Less Way may prove to be a safe and useful weight loss regimen. Importantly, it is also a sound plan for keeping the weight off. Of course, keeping calories to a reasonable level is still, and always will be, important, and it will always be the foundation of weight loss regimens. To boost the weight loss benefits of the AGE-Less Way, sample menus below provide about 1,600 calories per day. To suit your personal weight management goals, you may adjust calories by increasing or decreasing portions of the foods listed.

How many calories do you need? There are many mathematical formulas designed to estimate calorie needs, but most people need somewhere between 13 to 15 calories per pound to maintain their desired body weight. Very active people may need more calories and very sedentary people may need less. Many online calorie calculators are available. A good place to start is http://www.healthfinder.gov. Type "calorie calculator" into the search box to find links where you can estimate your calorie needs.

Six Weeks of AGE-Less Menus

The AGE-Less Way shows that we can reduce AGEs, have a complete meal, and eat it joyfully. Here we offer six weeks of sample menus featuring AGE-Less recipes from this book, as well as meal and snack suggestions that can be quickly assembled using foods that are widely available in grocery stores. You will find plenty of family favorites that even kids will love. Meat loaf, spaghetti and meatballs, stews, skillet dinners, sandwiches, omelets, puddings, and many other home-style comfort foods all work well on the AGE-Less Way.

The intent of these menus is not to present a regimented "diet" to which you should strictly adhere to, but to demonstrate tasty and creative meal planning possibilities. Use these ideas as you begin your AGE-Less path and let them serve as inspiration for your own meal makeovers, using the AGE-Less principles outlined in this book. These menus provide about 1,600 calories per day, so you may need to adjust portions to suit your personal nutrition goals. Note that portions sizes for recipes listed within the menus are for one serving unless otherwise noted.

Week 1

Breakfast	Lunch	Snacks	Dinner
Peach-Almond smoothie - Blend 1/2 cup low-fat milk, 1/2 cup light vanilla yogurt, 3/4 cup diced frozen peaches, 2 Tbsp raw almonds, and sugar substitute (optional) until smooth. Coffee/tea	Spicy Egg Salad Sandwich (p. 158) Cup of vegetable soup Tangerine	6 ounces light yogurt 3/4 cup grapes 1/4 cup raw pumpkin seeds	Chicken Dijon (p. 195) Served over 3/4 cup brown rice 1 1/2 cups steamed vegetable medley with 1 tsp olive oil and parsley Lemon Tapioca Pudding (p. 274)
Oatmeal (1 cup cooked) topped with 1 1/2 tbsp walnuts and 1/2 cup fresh berries 1 cup low-fat milk Coffee/tea	Chipotle Chicken Salad (p. 177) 1 oz. baked tortilla chips Fresh plum	Low-fat mozzarella cheese stick Medium fresh pear 3 Tbsp raw sunflower seeds	Mediterranean Baked Fish (p. 207) Served over 2/3 cup whole wheat couscous Broiled Asparagus & Onions (p. 236) 1/2 cup sugar-free pudding
Breakfast Banana Split - 1/2 banana (split open), topped with 6 oz. light vanilla yogurt, 1/2 cup blueberries, 1/4 cup low-fat granola, and 1 Tbsp walnuts Coffee/tea	Salmon Salad Nicoise (p. 185) Wedges of whole grain pita bread (1 oz) 1/2 cup sugar-free pudding	1 cup low-fat milk 2 Tbsp raw almonds Tangerine 1/2 oz. dark chocolate	Pork tenderloin with Sour Cream Sauce (p. 232) 1/2 medium baked acorn squash 1 cup steamed Brussels sprouts 2 tsp margarine Steamed Apples (p. 271)
Breakfast bagel - scrambled egg and 3/4 oz. light cheddar cheese in a 2-ounce whole grain bagel Fresh mixed fruit cup Coffee/tea	1 1/4 cups Savory Lentil Soup (p. 139) 1 cup fresh vegetables with 2 Tbsp light blue cheese dressing 6 oz. light yogurt	Low-fat mozzarella cheese stick Fresh plum	Spaghetti & Meatballs (p. 222) 3 cups garden Salad with 1 Tbsp Italian dressing 1/2 cup low-fat ice cream with 1/2 cup raspberries and 1 1/2 tbsp walnuts
Shredded Wheat cereal (1 cup) with 1 cup low-fat milk, 1/4 cup each blueberries and sliced bananas Coffee/tea	Couscous Shrimp Salad (p. 186) 3/4 cup fresh grapes	1 cup low-fat milk or low-fat latte 1 slice Oatmeal Banana Bread (p. 264) 3 Tbsp raw pumpkin seeds	1 1/2 cups Fasolada (Greek white bean soup) (p. 140) Whole grain roll (1 oz.) Spinach salad (2 cups) with sliced pears (1/3 cup), 1 tbsp each walnuts, dried cranberries, light feta cheese, and light balsamic dressing
Southwestern-Style Egg (p. 124) Fresh fruit cup 1 cup low-fat milk Coffee/tea	Mediterranean Tuna Wrap (p. 159) 3/4 cup Greek Broccoli Salad (p. 243)	3/4 cup bran flake cereal 1/2 banana 3/4 cup low-fat milk 3 Tbsp raw sunflower seeds	Cajun Meatloaf (p. 221) 1 cup steamed green beans with 1/2 tsp margarine and 1 Tbsp sliced almonds Smashed Potatoes with Garlic & Chives (p. 238) Lemon Parfait – 1/2 cup light lemon yogurt layered with 1/2 cup blackberries

2 slices Buttermilk French Toast (p. 130) Topped with 1/3 cup warm low-sugar apple pie filling (canned) Vegetarian sausage (1 1/2 oz) 1 cup low-fat milk Coffee/tea	Chicken & Broccoli Pasta Salad (p. 178) 3/4 cup diced mango	Citrus Cream Float – place 1/2 cup light vanilla ice cream in an 8-ounce wine glass and fill with 1/2 cup orange juice. 2 Tbsp raw almonds	Foil-Baked Fish with Summer Vegetables (p. 208) Served over 2/3 cup quinoa or whole wheat couscous Colorful Chopped Salad (p. 244) 1/2 oz. dark chocolate

Week 2

Breakfast	Lunch	Snack	Dinner
Strawberry smoothie – blenderize 1/2 cup light vanilla yogurt, 1/2 cup low-fat milk, 1 1/4 cups frozen strawberries, and 2 Tbsp walnuts or almonds Coffee/tea	Veggie burger on whole grain bun with 1/2 oz. light cheddar cheese, lettuce, tomato, and onion Cup of tomato soup	Apple Bran Muffin (p. 135) 1 cup low-fat milk	Skillet Beef Stroganoff (p. 227) Spinach Salad - 2 cups spinach; 1/4 cup mandarin oranges; 1 slice red onion; 1 1/2 Tbsp each walnuts, light mozzarella cheese, and light balsamic dressing. Pudding Parfait – layer 1/2 cup sugar-free pudding with 1/3 cup light cherry pie filling
Apricot-Almond Muesli (p. 126) Coffee/tea	Layered Seafood Salad (p. 179) Wedges of whole grain pita bred (1 oz.)	6 oz. light yogurt Medium apple 2 Tbsp raw pumpkin seeds	Black Bean Quesadilla (p. 160) Citrus-Avocado Salad (p. 248) 1 oz. dark chocolate
Frittata Primavera (p. 119) Mini whole grain bagel with 2 Tbsp Yogurt-Raisin-Walnut Spread (p. 263) Fresh fruit cup Coffee/tea	Chicken Salad Sandwich made with 1/2 cup Lemon-Herb Chicken Salad (p. 171), 1/4 cup avocado slices, 1/3 cup sprouts, and whole grain bread 3/4 cup grapes	1/3 cup hummus with 1 cup celery and carrot sticks Low-fat latte	Cod with Tomatoes & Capers (p. 212) Served over 1/2 cup whole grain angel hair pasta 1 cup zucchini & onions sautéed with 1 tsp olive oil and garlic 6 oz. light key lime yogurt layered with 1/2 cup raspberries and 1 Tbsp sliced almonds
Oatmeal (made from 1/2 cup dry) topped with 1/2 cup canned light pears and 2 tbsp walnuts 1 cup low-fat milk Coffee/tea	Shrimp Gazpacho (p. 147) 1/3 cup hummus with wedges of whole grain pita bread (1 oz.) Fresh plum	1 cup fresh cherries 6 ounces light yogurt with 2 Tbsp low-fat granola Hard-boiled egg	Chicken & Vegetables en Papillote (p. 196) Served over 1/2 cup brown rice Cucumber & Tomato Salad (p. 248) Moist Mocha Fudge Cake (p. 269)
Breakfast sandwich - mini whole grain bagel with one egg (scrambled in cooking spray), 3/4 oz. light cheddar cheese, and 1 slice vegetarian bacon Mixed fresh fruit cup Coffee/tea	Whole grain pita (2 oz) filled with Boston lettuce and 1 cup Chicken Salad with Grapes & Walnuts (p. 175) 1 cup baby carrots 6 ounces light yogurt	Medium apple Mozzarella cheese stick 2 Tbsp raw sunflower seeds	Cajun Shrimp Boil (p. 205) Green Bean & Grape Tomato Salad (p. 249) 1 oz. dark chocolate

Egg & Potato Skillet (p. 123) Mini whole grain bagel with 1 tsp margarine Grapefruit half Coffee/tea/ milk	Dilled Salmon Salad (p. 181) 1 kiwi fruit 6 oz. light yogurt	Cocoa-Banana Muffin (p. 134) 1 cup low-fat milk 2 Tbsp raw almonds	2 Soft Tacos (p. 229) Southwestern Cabbage Salad (p. 250) 1 cup honeydew melon
Portabella Mushroom Omelet (p. 117) Mini whole grain bagel with 2 tbsp Yogurt-Raisin-Walnut Spread (p. 263) Fresh fruit cup Coffee/tea	Fruited Chicken & Rice Salad (p. 172) 6 ounces light yogurt	Strawberry Gelato (p. 279) 2 Tbsp walnuts	Pasta with Shrimp & Scallops Arrabbiata (p. 213). 1 1/2 cups broccoli, cauliflower, and carrots sautéed with 1 tsp olive oil 1 oz. dark chocolate

Week 3

Breakfast	Lunch	Snack	Dinner
Poached egg on whole grain toast 1 cup fresh melon 1 cup low-fat milk Coffee/tea	Tuna sandwich (1/2 can) on 2 slices whole grain bread, with 1/4 cup avocado slices, 1/3 cup sprouts, and nonfat mayo Cup of minestrone soup 6 oz. light yogurt	1/4 cup Creamy Artichoke Spread (p. 259) With 1 cup carrot and celery sticks Fresh plum 3 Tbsp walnuts	Chicken & Potato Pot Pie (p. 203) Spinach & Mushroom Salad (2 cups) with 1 slice red onion, 1/4 cup grape tomatoes, and 1 1/2 Tbsp each reduced-fat cheddar, and light ranch dressing Strawberry Mousse (p. 278)
Mixed berry smoothie - Blenderize 3/4 cup low-fat milk, 1/2 cup light vanilla yogurt, 1 cup frozen mixed berries, 1 1/2 tablespoons walnuts, 1 Tbsp oat bran, and sugar substitute until smooth. Coffee/tea	1 1/2 cups Beef & Barley Soup (p. 145) Half veggie sandwich - 1 slice whole grain bread, 1 oz. light Swiss cheese, fresh spinach, carrots, onion, and 2 Tbsp marinated artichoke hearts Fresh plum	1 cup low-fat milk or sugar-free chocolate milk 2 Tbsp raw almonds Fresh nectarine	Saffron Chicken & Orzo (p. 200) 1 1/2 cups steamed vegetable medley with 1 tsp margarine Key Lime Panna Cotta (p. 273)
1 cup hot multigrain cereal with 1/2 cup canned diced pears and 2 tbsp walnuts 1 cup low-fat milk Coffee/tea	Mediterranean Chopped Salad (p. 176) Wedges of whole grain pita bread (1 oz.) Fresh mixed fruit cup	1 slice Oatmeal Banana Bread (p. 264) 1 cup low-fat milk 2 Tbsp raw sunflower seeds	Steamed Fish with Ginger Sauce (p. 206) Vegetable Fried Rice (p. 240) 3/4 cup fresh orange sections drizzled with 1 tsp honey and 1 Tbsp sliced almonds
Sausage & Egg Burrito (p. 125) 6 ounces low-sodium vegetable juice cocktail Coffee/tea	Tabbouleh Tuna Salad (p. 184) Fresh mixed fruit cup	6 oz. light vanilla yogurt 2 Tbsp raw pumpkin seeds with 2 Tbsp raisins	Bodacious Burger (p. 157) in a whole grain bun with lettuce, tomato, and onion Boiled corn on the cob with 1/2 tsp margarine 3/4 cup low-fat broccoli slaw 1 oz. dark chocolate

Oatmeal (cooked from 1/2 cup dry) with 1/2 sliced banana and 2 tbsp pecans or walnuts 1 cup low-fat milk Coffee/tea/milk	Couscous Chicken Salad (p. 174) Fresh peach 2 Tbsp raw almonds	Hard boiled egg 6 oz. vegetable juice cocktail Tangerine	1 1/2 cups Fiesta Chili (p. 142) Topped with 2 tbsp shredded light cheddar cheese 3/4 cup coleslaw made with light ranch dressing 1/2 cup fruit sorbet
2 slices Buttermilk French Toast (p. 130) With 1/3 cup Warm Strawberry Sauce (p. 133) 1 1/2 oz. vegetarian sausage 1 cup low-fat milk Coffee/tea	Spinach Pita Pizza (p. 162) Mixed green salad (2 cups) with 1 Tbsp light vinaigrette dressing	Blueberry-Banana Smoothie – blend 1/2 cup each frozen blueberries, frozen sliced bananas, light vanilla yogurt, and 3/4 cup low-fat milk until smooth. 3 Tbsp raw almonds	Whitefish with Tomatoes, Peas & Parsley Sauce (p. 211) 1 cup steamed cauliflower Whole grain roll 1 tsp margarine Citrus Poached Pear (p. 272)
Spinach & Potato Frittata (p. 120) 1 piece whole grain toast with 1 tsp margarine Fresh mixed fruit cup Coffee/tea	1 1/2 cups Meatball Soup (p. 146) Half veggie sandwich – whole grain bread, 1 oz. low-fat mozzarella, cucumbers, tomato, red onion, carrots, spinach, and 1 tsp light Italian dressing.	6 oz. light yogurt Fresh peach 3 Tbsp raw almonds	Pasta with Shrimp & Broccoli (p. 214) 2 1/2 cups garden salad with 1 Tbsp each black olives, mozzarella, and light olive oil vinaigrette Cherry-Berry Delight (p. 275)

Week 4

Breakfast	Lunch	Snack	Dinner
Poached egg on whole wheat toast 1 cup low-fat milk Fresh mixed fruit cup Coffee/tea	Very Veggie Sandwich (p. 163) Medium apple	1/3 cup Spicy Garbanzo Spread (p. 260) 1 cup fresh cut vegetables 1/4 cup raw pumpkin seeds	Saucy Stuffed Cabbage (p. 228) 1 1/2 cups steamed broccoli, cauliflower, and carrots with 1 tsp olive oil and dill Pudding Parfait – layer 1/2 cup sugar-free pudding with 1/2 cup sliced bananas
Oatmeal (cooked from 1/2 cup dry) with 1/2 cup fresh berries and 1 1/2 tbsp sliced almonds 1 cup low-fat milk Coffee/tea	1 cup Lemon-Herb Chicken Salad (p. 171) Served over 2 cups mixed baby salad greens with 1 Tbsp light vinaigrette dressing Whole grain pita wedges (1 oz.) 1 cup cantaloupe	Half veggie sandwich made with whole grain bread, 1 oz. low-fat mozzarella cheese, salad greens, and 1/4 cup marinated artichoke hearts Tangerine 3 Tbsp raw sunflower seeds	Roasted Ratatouille (p. 234) served over 1/2 cup brown rice or couscous 1 cup green beans sautéed with mushrooms and 1 tsp olive oil Dark Chocolate Mousse (p. 277)

Apple Bran Muffin (p. 135) Hard boiled egg 1 cup low-fat milk Coffee/tea	Chicken Tortilla Soup (p. 151) Fresh vegetables with 2 tbsp light ranch dressing 1 cup fresh melon	Mini whole grain bagel with 1/4 cup Yogurt-Raisin-Walnut Spread (p. 263) Fresh plum	Penne with Spicy Shrimp & Artichokes (p. 215) Spinach salad with 1 Tbsp Italian dressing Parfait - layer 1/2 cup sugar-free pudding with 1/4 cup canned light cherry pie filling and 2 Tbsp sliced raw almonds
Poached Egg with Salmon & Tomato-Caper Salsa (p. 115) Fresh fruit cup 1 cup low-fat milk Coffee/tea	Cup of minestrone soup Tuna pita - 1/2 can water-packed tuna, 1 cup salad mix, 1 Tbsp Italian dressing, whole grain pita Tangerine	Cocoa-Banana Muffin (p. 134) 1 cup low-fat milk 2 Tbsp walnuts	1 1/4 cups Harvest Black Bean Chili (p. 141) with 2 Tbsp light Monterey Jack cheese 1 cup cooked cabbage with 1 tsp olive oil 1/2 cup light yogurt with 1/2 cup sliced strawberries
Whole grain pita pocket (1 oz) filled with 1/4 cup scrambled egg substitute and 1 oz. vegetarian sausage Fresh fruit cup 1 cup low-fat milk Coffee/tea	Orzo Crab Salad (p. 182) served over 2 cups mixed baby salad greens with 1 Tbsp vinaigrette dressing Cup of vegetable soup	6 oz. light yogurt 1 kiwi fruit 1/4 cup raw sunflower seeds	Beef Stew Provencal (p. 143) served over 3/4 cup low-fat mashed potatoes 2 1/2 cups garden salad with 2 Tbsp light blue cheese dressing Razzleberry Gelatin (p. 276)
Hot & Hearty Oats (p. 127) topped with 1/2 cup fresh berries and 2 Tbsp walnuts 1 cup low-fat milk Coffee/tea	1 1/2 cups Chicken, Barley & Corn Chowder (p. 150) Fresh cut vegetables with 2 tbsp light blue cheese dressing 3/4 cup fresh cherries	6 oz. light vanilla yogurt layered with 1/2 cup fresh or canned light peaches and 2 Tbsp low-fat granola	Seafood Stew with Fire-Roasted Tomatoes (p. 149) 1 oz. multigrain French bread 2 1/2 cups garden salad with 1 Tbsp Italian dressing 1 oz. dark chocolate
Caramelized Onion & Pepper Omelet (p. 118) 1 slice whole grain toast with 1 tsp margarine 1 cup cantaloupe 1 cup low-fat milk Coffee/tea	Whole grain wrap filled with grilled portabella mushroom, 1 oz. fresh mozzarella cheese, fresh spinach, tomato, onion, and 1 1/2 tsp balsamic dressing Fresh nectarine	1/3 cup Spicy Garbanzo Spread (p. 260) with 1 cup carrot and celery sticks 3 Tbsp raw pumpkin seeds	Chicken Florentine (p. 201) Green salad topped with julienne beets, mandarin oranges and 1 tbsp each light balsamic dressing and light feta cheese Whole grain roll 1/2 cup light vanilla yogurt with 1/2 cup sliced strawberries and 1 tbsp sliced almonds

Week 5

Breakfast	Lunch	Snack	Dinner
6 oz low-fat Greek-style yogurt layered with 1/2 cup fresh blueberries, 1/4 cup orange sections, and 3 Tbsp low-fat granola Coffee/tea	Spicy Garbanzo Wrap (p. 164) Fresh plum Low-fat mozzarella cheese stick	1 slice Oatmeal Banana Bread (p. 264) 1 cup low-fat milk 2 Tbsp walnuts	Crab cakes with Roasted Red Pepper Sauce (p. 217) Boiled corn on the cob with 1 tsp margarine 1 1/2 cups steamed vegetable medley tossed with 1 tsp Basil Pesto (p. 257) 2 broiled pineapple slices with 1/2 cup light vanilla ice cream and 1 Tbsp sliced almonds
Breakfast sandwich made with whole grain English muffin, scrambled egg, and 3/4 oz. light cheddar cheese Fresh mixed fruit cup Coffee/tea	1 1/2 cups Chunky Potato Soup (p. 153) 1/2 low-fat chicken salad sandwich	Tangerine smoothie – blend 1 cup frozen seedless tangerine sections, 1/2 cup light vanilla yogurt, 1/2 cup low-fat milk, and sugar substitute (optional) until smooth	Chili-Macaroni (p. 224) 1 cup sautéed vegetable medley with 1 tsp margarine and parsley 2 cups mixed green salad with 1 Tbsp light ranch dressing 1/2 cup sugar-free pudding with 1/2 cup raspberries and 1 1/2 Tbsp walnuts
Mocha-Banana Smoothie (p. 136) Hard boiled egg Coffee/tea	Tuna Salad with Pasta & Roasted Red Peppers (p. 187) Cup of vegetable soup	Fresh pear 6 oz light yogurt 1/4 cup raw sunflower seeds	1 1/2 cups Creamy Asparagus Soup (p. 155) Roasted Red Pepper Quesadilla (p. 161) 1 oz. dark chocolate
1/2 cup fresh or canned light apricots layered with 6 oz. light vanilla yogurt and 1/4 cup low-fat granola Coffee/tea	Sesame Noodle Salad (p. 189) 3/4 cup fresh pineapple	1 slice Zucchini Spice Bread (p. 266) 1 cup nonfat or low-fat milk 2 Tbsp walnuts	Greek-Style Skillet Dinner (p. 225) 1 cup steamed green beans with 1 Tbsp sliced almonds 1 cup Greek Chopped Salad (p. 245) 3/4 cup light vanilla ice cream with 1/2 cup fresh raspberries
1 1/4 cups Shredded Wheat Cereal with 1/2 cup sliced banana 1 cup low-fat milk Coffee/tea	Whole wheat wrap filled with 1/2 cup Artichoke Chicken Salad (p. 172) and mixed baby salad greens Cup of lentil soup	Orange 1 oz. low-fat mozzarella cheese stick 1/4 cup raw pumpkin seeds	Asian-Style Steamed Chicken with Cilantro Sauce (p. 194) 1 cup Fried Rice with Spinach & Sesame (p. 241) 1 cup steamed baby carrots with 1 tsp margarine 3/4 cup fresh pineapple
Filled Pancakes with Fruit Sauce (p. 130) 1 1/2 oz. vegetarian sausage 1 cup low-fat milk Coffee/tea	Shrimp Cobb Salad (p. 180) Wedges of whole grain pita bread (1 oz.) Cup of minestrone soup	1/2 cup seedless red grapes layered with 6 oz. low-fat Greek-style yogurt and 2 tbsp walnuts	White Bean Cassoulet (p. 233) 1 1/2 cups steamed vegetable medley with 1 tsp Basil Pesto (p. 257) Sliced fresh tomatoes and cucumbers with 1 tsp Italian dressing Grilled Plums with Goat Cheese (p. 271)
Hot Buckwheat Cereal with Apples and Walnuts (p. 128) Coffee/tea	Pita & Portabella Panini (p. 166) Cup of lentil soup 1/2 cup baby carrots with 1 Tbsp light blue cheese dressing	Hard-boiled egg 6 oz. V-8 juice 3 Tbsp raw sunflower seeds Fresh plum	Moroccan Meatballs with Sweet Onion Sauce (p. 198) Cauliflower & Couscous Pilaf (p. 242) 1 cup steamed Brussels sprouts with 1 tsp olive oil

Week 6

Breakfast	Lunch	Snack	Dinner
Egg white omelet with spinach, scallions, and 2 Tbsp light cheddar cheese Mini whole grain bagel with 1 tsp margarine 1/2 cup orange juice 1 cup low-fat milk Coffee/tea	Artichoke Chicken Salad (p. 172) served over 2 cups mixed baby salad greens Cup of white bean soup Plum	Cool Cappuccino Frappe (p. 267) Fresh pear 2 Tbsp raw almonds	Pork Carnitas (p. 231) with 2 warm corn tortillas, 1/4 cup avocado slices, lettuce, and salsa 1 cup zucchini and onions sautéed in 1 tsp olive oil 1 1/2 cups watermelon
Tropical Fruit Smoothie - Blend 1/2 cup each frozen pineapple chunks, frozen sliced banana, low-fat milk, and light vanilla yogurt, with 2 Tbsp sliced almonds, and sugar substitute (optional) until smooth. Coffee/tea	BLT sandwich – 4 slices vegetarian bacon, 2 slices multigrain bread, lettuce, tomato, low-fat mayonnaise. 3/4 cup low-fat coleslaw Medium apple	Low-fat latte 1 slice Zucchini Spice Bread (p. 266) 3 Tbsp raw pumpkin seeds	Oven-Braised Turkey Breast with Gravy (p. 204) 1/2 cup mashed potatoes (low-fat recipe) Whole grain roll 1 1/2 cups steamed vegetable medley with 1 tsp margarine 1 oz dark chocolate
1 cup Raisin Bran cereal 1 cup low-fat milk Grapefruit half Coffee/tea	Great Garbanzo Salad (p. 190) Wedges of whole grain pita bread (1 oz.) Orange	1/2 veggie sandwich – 1 slice whole grain bread, 1 ounce low-fat cheese, marinated artichoke hearts, spinach, and tomato 1 cup fresh strawberries 3 Tbsp raw almonds	Oven Braised Pot Roast (p. 223) Steamed new potatoes and baby carrots (1/2 cup each) 3/4 cup cooked collard greens 1/2 cup sugar-free pudding
Egg Quesadilla with Spinach & Cheese (p. 116) 6 oz. low-sodium vegetable juice Coffee/tea	Cannellini Tuna Salad (p. 188) Cup of tomato soup 1 cup grapes 1/2 oz. dark chocolate	6 oz. light yogurt Kiwi fruit 3 Tbsp walnuts	Unfried Falafel (p. 167) 1 cup Garden Fresh Tabbouleh (p. 246) 1 cup fresh melon
Quinoa with Bananas, Raisins, & Pecans (p. 129) 1 cup low-fat milk Coffee/tea	1/2 whole grain pita filled with 1/3 cup low-fat egg salad, 2 Tbsp grated carrots, and 1/3 cup sprouts 1 cup Barley Salad with Broccoli, Corn, & Tomatoes (p. 247)	Low-fat mozzarella cheese stick Tangerine 1/4 cup raw pumpkin seeds	Summertime Crab Salad (p. 183) Cup of vegetable soup Whole grain roll Cherry Gelato (p. 280)

Cauliflower & Feta Cheese Frittata (p. 122) mini whole grain bagel with 1 tsp margarine Mixed fresh fruit cup Coffee/tea	1 1/2 cups Home-Style Chicken Soup (p. 152) 1 cup fresh cut vegetables with 2 tbsp low-fat ranch dressing 6 oz. light yogurt	1 cup low-fat milk Apple Bran Muffin (p. 135) 2 Tbsp walnuts	Flavorful Fried Rice (p. 219) Asian Slaw with Almonds (p. 251) Fresh nectarine
3 Whole Grain Hotcakes (p. 132) with 1/3 cup Warm Strawberry Sauce (p. 133) 1 1/2 oz. vegetarian sausage patty 1 cup low-fat milk Coffee/tea	1 cup Colorful Lentil Salad (p. 191) Cup of vegetable soup Low-fat mozzarella cheese stick	1/2 cup Roasted Eggplant Spread (p. 262) Wedges of whole grain pita bread (1 ounce) 1/2 cup baby carrots	Poached fish (5 oz) with 1/4 cup Chilean Pebre Sauce (p. 254) 1 cup black beans & brown rice, with 1 tsp olive oil 1 cup sautéed zucchini, corn, red peppers, with 1 tsp margarine Cappuccino Granita (p. 281)

Appendix
AGE Content in Selected Food Items

FOOD ITEMS	AGE kilounits

Meat and meat substitutes

Poultry

Chicken, skinless breast, broiled 15 min, 3 oz	5200
Chicken, skinless breast, marinated, George Foreman grill 5 min, 3 oz	890
Chicken, breast skinless, poached or simmered in soup/stew (with water or broth), 3 oz.	940
Chicken breast, skinless, poached or simmered in soup/stew (with addition of acidic ingredients such as lemon, wine, or tomatoes), 3 oz.	580
Chicken, skinless breast, slow cooker, 3 hours, high power, with wine and broth, 3 oz.	740
Chicken breast baked in foil packet, 3 oz (see Chicken Dijon recipe, page 195)	890
Turkey, roasted, 3 oz	4000
Turkey breast, oven-braised with white wine (see Oven-Braised Turkey Breast recipe, page 204), 3 oz	774

Beef

Beef steak broiled, 3 oz	6600
Beef, roast, 3 oz.	5465

Beef, roast, lean, oven-braised in red wine and broth
(see Oven-Braised Pot Roast recipe, page 223), 3 oz.   1065

Beef hamburger, 3 oz   2400

Beef hamburger, 93% lean (see Bodacious Burger recipe,
page 157)   1110

Beef meatballs   3220

Beef meatballs, lower-fat recipe (see Spaghetti & Meatballs
recipe, page 222), 3 oz   1220

Beef, meatloaf, lower-fat recipe (see Cajun Meatloaf recipe,
page 221), 3 oz.   930

Beef, 93% lean, taco filling (see Soft Taco recipe,
page 229) 3 oz.   940

Beef, stewed, 3 oz.   2200

Beef, lean, stewed with tomatoes and red wine,
(see Beef Stew Provencal recipe, page 143) 3 oz.   990

Pork

Bacon, fried, 2 strips   11000

Pork ribs, Chinese take out, 3 oz   4000

Pork tenderloin, braised in broth and wine (see Pork
Tenderloin With Sour Cream Sauce recipe, page 232), 3 oz.   1025

Pork Carnitas, braised in beer (see Pork Carnitas recipe,
page 231), 3 oz   795

Fish and seafood

Crabmeat, fried (take out), 3 oz   3030

Crab cake, low-fat recipe (see Crab Cakes with Roasted
Red Pepper Sauce recipe, page 217), 3 oz.   765

Crabmeat, boiled, 3 oz.   410

Salmon, poached or steamed, 3 oz.   1330

Salmon, canned, 3 oz.   825

Tuna, canned in oil, 3 oz   1600

Tuna, canned in water, 3 oz.   410

Flounder, baked in foil packet (see Foil-Baked Fish with
Summer Vegetables recipe, page 208), 3 oz   455

Flounder, baked with tomatoes and wine (see Mediterranean
Baked Fish recipe, page 207), 3 oz.   410
Flounder, covered skillet, medium heat, 3 min/side,
cooking spray, 3 oz.   655
Shrimp, simmered in stew with tomatoes (see Seafood
Stew with Fire-Roasted Tomatoes, page 149), 3 oz.   380
Shrimp marinated in light balsamic salad dressing,
broiled 2 min/side, 3 oz.   540

Legumes & Soy

Beans, red kidney, canned, 3 oz.   190
Hummus, ½ cup   700
Tofu, raw, 3 oz.   710
Tofu, broiled, 3 oz.   3700
Veggie burger, cooking spray, 2 oz.   85
Vegetarian bacon, microwaved 2 min at high power until crisp, 1 oz.   430
Vegetarian sausage link, pan cover, cooking spray, 1 oz.   240

Eggs

Egg (whole), fried, 1 large   1240
Egg, scrambled or omelet, cooking spray, 1 oz   30
Egg, poached, 5 min, 1 oz.   30

Cheese

American, 1 oz.   2605
American, low fat, 1 oz.   1210
Brie, 1 oz.   1680
Cream cheese, 1 Tbsp   1470
Cheddar, 1 oz.   1660
Cheddar, reduced-fat, 1 oz.   740
Cottage, low-fat, 1/2 cup   1733
Feta, 1 oz.   2530
Mozzarella, reduced-fat, 1 oz.   505
Ricotta, part skim, 1/4 cup   1160
Parmesan, 2 teaspoons   845

Nuts & Seeds

Almonds, blanched, slivered, 1 oz.	1645
Almonds, roasted, 1 oz.	1995
Cashews, raw, 1 oz.	2020
Cashews, roasted, 1 oz.	2940
Chestnut, raw, 1 oz.	820
Chestnut, roasted, 1 oz.	1610
Peanuts, roasted, 1 oz.	2220
Peanut butter, 1 oz.	2255
Pumpkin seeds, raw, 1 oz.	560
Sunflower seeds, raw, 1 oz.	755
Sunflower seeds, roasted, 1 oz.	1410

Fats and oils

Avocado, 1 oz.	475
Butter, 1 Tbsp	1890
Coconut cream, 1 Tbsp	140
Cream, heavy, 1 Tbsp	325
Margarine, 1 Tbsp	540
Mayonnaise, 1 Tbsp	1400
Mayonnaise, low-fat, 1 Tbsp	330
Mayonnaise, nonfat, 1 Tbsp	30
Olives, ripe, 1 oz.	500
Salad dressing, 1 Tbsp	107
Canola oil, 1 Tbsp	885
Corn oil, 1 Tbsp	1455
Olive oil, 1 Tbsp	450
Sesame seed oil (non-toasted), 1 Tbsp	390

Breads

Bagel, 1 oz.	35
Bagel, toasted, 1 oz.	50
Biscuit, fast food, 1 oz.	440
Biscuit, refrigerator, baked, 1 oz.	400
Bread, sandwich-type, 1 oz.	35

Bread, Greek, hard, 1 oz.	45
Bread, Greek, hard, toasted, 1 oz.	180
Bread, Greek, soft, 1 oz.	35
Bread, pita, 1 oz.	15
Croissant, 1 oz.	335

Cereals & Breakfast Foods

Cereal, Bran flakes, 1 oz.	10
Cereal, Corn flakes, 1 oz	70
Cereal, Corn flakes, frosted, 1 oz.	130
Cereal, Fiber One, 1 oz.	420
Cereal, Granola, 1 oz.	130
Cereal, Oatmeal, instant dry, 1 oz	5
Cereal, Puffed wheat, 1 oz.	5
Cereal, Rice Krispies, 1 oz	600
Cereal, Shredded wheat, frosted, 1 oz.	65
French toast, frozen, microwaved, 1 oz.	180
Muffin, bran, low-fat, 1 oz.	220
Pancake, from mix, 1 oz.	250
Waffle, frozen, toasted, 1 oz	675

Grains & Starches

Corn, canned, 3 oz.	20
Pasta, cooked 8 min, 3 oz.	110
Pasta, cooked 12 min, 3 oz.	240
Potato, sweet, roasted 1 hr, 3 oz.	70
Potato, white, boiled, 3 oz.	20
Rice, cooked, 3 oz.	20

Fruits

Apple, raw, 3 oz.	15
Apple, baked, 3 oz	45

Banana, 3 oz	10
Cantaloupe, 3 oz.	20
Coconut, sweetened, flaked, 1 oz.	180
Dates, 1 oz.	20
Plums, dried, 1 oz.	50
Raisins, 1 oz	36
Fruit juice, 8 oz	10

Vegetables

Asparagus, broiled, low-fat recipe, 3 oz.	200
Cucumber, 3 oz	31
Carrots, 3 oz	10
Green beans, canned, 3 oz.	20
Mushrooms, Portabella, roasted, low-fat recipe, 3 oz (see recipe, page 117)	210
Tomatoes, 3 oz	25
Vegetable juice, V8, 8 oz	5

Crackers/snacks

Cheeze curls, 1 oz.	965
Chex mix, 1 oz.	350
Chips, corn, 1 oz.	270
Chips, potato, 1 oz	865
Chips, potato, baked, 1 oz.	135
Cracker, goldfish, 1 oz.	650
Cracker, graham, 1 oz.	430
Cracker, melba toast, 1 oz.	270
Cracker, oyster, 1 oz.	510
Cracker, rice cake, 1 oz.	40
Cracker, saltine, 1 oz.	280
Cracker, sandwich-type, club + cheddar, 1 oz.	550
Cracker, toasted wheat, 1 oz.	275

Popcorn, microwaved,no-fat, 1 oz.	10
Pretzel, 1 oz.	530

Sweets*

Bar, granola, chocolate chunk, soft, 1 oz	150
Bar, granola, peanut butter & chocolate chunk, 1 oz.	950
Bar, rice krispy treat, 1 oz.	575
Bread, banana, low-fat (see Oatmeal Banana Bread recipe, page 264), 1 oz	124
Candy, chocolate, dark, 1 oz.	535
Candy, chocolate-covered raisins, 1 oz.	60
Candy, chocolate-peanut butter cup, 1 oz.	1030
Cookie, biscotti, 1 oz	970
Cookie, chocolate chip,1 oz	500
Cookie, fortune, 1 oz.	30
Cookie, Greek wedding, nut, 1 oz.	290
Cookie, meringue, homemade, 1 oz.	240
Cookie, Oreo, 1 oz	530
Cookie, vanilla wafer,1 oz.	150
Donut, chocolate iced, crème filled, 1 oz	540
Donut, chocolate glazed, 1 oz.	420
Fruit pot, frozen, 2 oz.	10
Gelatin, strawberry, 4 oz	2
Scone, cinnamon, 1 oz.	237
Sorbet, 1/2 cup	5
Sweet roll, cinnamon swirl, 1 oz.	270

*Note that AGEs are listed per 1 oz. for most of the above foods, but actual serving size may be several ounces.

Milk & Milk Products

Cocoa packet, sugar free, prepared, 8 oz	510
Ice cream, vanilla, 8 oz	85

Soy, milk, 8 oz	80
Milk, whole (4% fat), 8 oz	10
Milk, fat free, 8 oz	5
Pudding, instant, fat-free, sugar-free, prepared, 1/2 cup	1
Pudding, snack pak, 1/2 cup	20
Yogurt, vanilla or fruit-flavored, 8 oz	10

Soups

Soup, beef or chicken bouillon, 1 cup	3
Soup, chicken noodle, 1 cup	5
Soup, Cream of Celery Soup, condensed, reduced-fat, 3 oz.	115
Soup, vegetable, 1 cup	5

Fast foods

Bacon Egg Cheese Biscuit, 1 serving	2290
Double Quarter Pounder with Cheese, 1 serving	18000
Big Mac, 1 serving	17100
Chicken nuggets, 6 nuggets	9100
Grilled Chicken Sandwich, 1 serving	5170
Fried fish sandwich, 1 serving	6030
Pizza, 3 oz	6825
Cheeseburger, 1 serving	3400
French fries, small pack	1000

* The AGE content in right column is expressed in AGE kilo units per serving of food and based on the measurement of carboxymethyl-lysine (CML) by ELISA, as published (adapted from: Uribarri, J., Woodruff, S., Goodman, S., Cai, W., Chen, X., Pyzik, R., Yong, A., Striker, G. E. and Vlassara, H., Advanced glycation end products in foods and a practical guide to their reduction in the diet, *J Am Diet Assoc*, 2010, 110: 911-916 e912.

REFERENCES BY CHAPTER

CHAPTER 1:

1 Amos, A. F., McCarty, D. J. and Zimmet, P., The rising global burden of diabetes and its complications: estimates and projections to the year 2010, Diabet Med, 1997, 14 Suppl 5: S1-85.

2 Drewnowski, A. and Specter, S. E., Poverty and obesity: the role of energy density and energy costs, Am J Clin Nutr, 2004, 79: 6-16.

3 Parthasarathy, S., Khan-Merchant, N., Penumetcha, M., Khan, B. V. and Santanam, N., Did the antioxidant trials fail to validate the oxidation hypothesis? Curr Atheroscler Rep, 2001, 3: 392-398.

4 Hutson, S., Experts Urge a More Measured Look at Antioxidants, Nature Medicine, 2008, 14: 795.

5 Finot, P. A., Historical perspective of the Maillard reaction in food science, Ann N Y Acad Sci, 2005, 1043: 1-8.

6 Maillard, L. C., Action des acides anines sur les sucres: formation des melanoidines par voie methodique., C R Acad Sci, 1912, 154: 1653-1671.

7 Koenig, R. J., Peterson, C.M., Jones, R.L., Saudek, C., Lehrman, M., Cerami, A., Correlation of glucose regulation and hemoglobin A1C., J. Bio. Chem., 1977, 252: 2992-2997.

8 Bunn, H. F., Shapiro, R., McManus, M., Garrick, L., McDonald, M. J., Gallop, P. M. and Gabbay, K. H., Structural heterogeneity of human hemoglobin A due to nonenzymatic glycosylation, J Biol Chem, 1979, 254: 3892-3898.

8   Bunn, H. F. and Higgins, P. J., Reaction of monosaccharides with proteins: possible evolutionary significance, Science, 1981, 213: 222-224.

9   Brownlee, M., Cerami, A. and Vlassara, H., Advanced glycosylation end products in tissue and the biochemical basis of diabetic complications, N Engl J Med, 1988, 318: 1315-1321.

10 Baynes, J. W. and Thorpe, S. R., Role of oxidative stress in diabetic complications: a new perspective on an old paradigm, Diabetes, 1999, 48: 1-9.

11 Monnier, V. M., Cerami, T., Nonenzymatic browning in vivo: possible process for aging of long-lived proteins., Science, 1981, 211: 491-493.

12 Sell, D. R., Lapolla, A., Odetti, P., Fogarty, J. and Monnier, V. M., Pentosidine formation in skin correlates with severity of complications in individuals with long-standing IDDM, Diabetes, 1992, 41: 1286-1292.

13 Vlassara, H., Bucala, R. and Striker, L., Pathogenic effects of advanced glycosylation: biochemical, biologic, and clinical implications for diabetes and aging, Lab Invest, 1994, 70: 138-151.

16 Koschinsky, T., He, C. J., Mitsuhashi, T., Bucala, R., Liu, C., Buenting, C., Heitmann, K. and Vlassara, H., Orally absorbed reactive glycation products (glycotoxins): an environmental risk factor in diabetic nephropathy, Proc Natl Acad Sci U S A, 1997, 94: 6474-6479.

17 Vlassara, H., Brownlee, M., Manogue, K. R., Dinarello, C. A. and Pasagian, A., Cachectin/TNF and IL-1 induced by glucose-modified proteins: role in normal tissue remodeling, Science, 1988, 240: 1546-1548.

18 Pollan, M., The Omnivore's Dilemma: A Natural History of Four Meals, New York, Penguin Press, 2006.

19 USDA, Major Trends in U.S. Food Supply, 1909-99, 2000.

20 Nestle, M., Real Food: What to Eat New York, North Point Press, 2006.

21 Willett, W. C., Diet and health: what should we eat?, Science, 1994, 264: 532-537.

CHAPTER 2:

1   Hu, F. B., Stampfer, M. J., Manson, J. E., Ascherio, A., Colditz, G. A., Speizer, F. E., Hennekens, C. H. and Willett, W. C., Dietary saturated fats and their food sources in relation to the risk of coronary heart disease in women, Am J Clin Nutr, 1999, 70: 1001-1008.

2   Stampfer, M. J., Hu, F. B., Manson, J. E., Rimm, E. B. and Willett, W. C., Primary prevention of coronary heart disease in women through diet and lifestyle, N Engl J Med, 2000, 343: 16-22.

3   Bernstein, A. M., Sun, Q., Hu, F. B., Stampfer, M. J., Manson, J. E. and Willett, W. C., Major dietary protein sources and risk of coronary heart disease in women, Circulation, 2010, 122: 876-883.

4   Halton, T. L., Willett, W. C., Liu, S., Manson, J. E., Stampfer, M. J. and Hu, F. B., Potato and french fry consumption and risk of type 2 diabetes in women, Am J Clin Nutr, 2006, 83: 284-290.

5   Sinha, R., Cross, A. J., Graubard, B. I., Leitzmann, M. F. and Schatzkin, A., Meat intake and mortality: a prospective study of over half a million people, Arch Intern Med, 2009, 169: 562-571.

6   Fox, C. S., Pencina, M. J., Meigs, J. B., Vasan, R. S., Levitzky, Y. S. and D'Agostino, R. B., Sr., Trends in the incidence of type 2 diabetes mellitus from the 1970s to the 1990s: the Framingham Heart Study, Circulation, 2006, 113: 2914-2918.

7   Ruderman, N., Chisholm, D., Pi-Sunyer, X. and Schneider, S., The metabolically obese, normal-weight individual revisited, Diabetes, 1998, 47: 699-713.

8   Wildman, R. P., Muntner, P., Reynolds, K., McGinn, A. P., Rajpathak, S., Wylie-Rosett, J. and Sowers, M. R., The obese without cardiometabolic risk factor clustering and the normal weight with cardiometabolic risk factor clustering: prevalence and correlates of 2 phenotypes among the US population (NHANES 1999-2004), Arch Intern Med, 2008, 168: 1617-1624.

9   Uribarri, J., Cai, W., Peppa, M., Goodman, S., Ferrucci, L., Striker, G. and Vlassara, H., Circulating glycotoxins and dietary

advanced glycation endproducts: two links to inflammatory response, oxidative stress, and aging, J Gerontol A Biol Sci Med Sci, 2007, 62: 427-433.

10 Huebschmann, A. G., Regensteiner, J. G., Vlassara, H. and Reusch, J. E., Diabetes and advanced glycoxidation end products, Diabetes Care, 2006, 29: 1420-1432.

11 Vlassara, H., Cai, W., Goodman, S., Pyzik, R., Yong, A., Chen, X., Zhu, L., Neade, T., Beeri, M., Silverman, J. M., Ferrucci, L., Tansman, L., Striker, G. E. and Uribarri, J., Protection against loss of innate defenses in adulthood by low advanced glycation end products (AGE) intake: role of the antiinflammatory AGE receptor-1, J Clin Endocrinol Metab, 2009, 94: 4483-4491.

12 Goldberg, T., Cai, W., Peppa, M., Dardaine, V., Baliga, B. S., Uribarri, J. and Vlassara, H., Advanced glycoxidation end products in commonly consumed foods, J Am Diet Assoc, 2004, 104: 1287-1291.

13 Uribarri, J., Woodruff, S., Goodman, S., Cai, W., Chen, X., Pyzik, R., Yong, A., Striker, G. E. and Vlassara, H., Advanced glycation end products in foods and a practical guide to their reduction in the diet, J Am Diet Assoc, 2010, 110: 911-916 e912.

14 van Dam, R. M., Willett, W. C., Rimm, E. B., Stampfer, M. J. and Hu, F. B., Dietary fat and meat intake in relation to risk of type 2 diabetes in men, Diabetes Care, 2002, 25: 417-424.

6 Levenstein, H., Paradox of Plenty: A Social History of Eating in Modern America, Berkeley, University of California Press, 2003.

CHAPTER 3:

1 Cai, W., Gao, Q. D., Zhu, L., Peppa, M., He, C. and Vlassara, H., Oxidative stress-inducing carbonyl compounds from common foods: novel mediators of cellular dysfunction, Mol Med, 2002, 8: 337-346.

2 Brands, C. M., Alink, G. M., van Boekel, M. A. and Jongen, W. M., Mutagenicity of heated sugar-casein systems: effect of the Maillard reaction, J Agric Food Chem, 2000, 48: 2271-2275.

3 Birlouez-Aragon, I., Saavedra, G., Tessier, F. J., Galinier, A., Ait-Ameur, L., Lacoste, F., Niamba, C. N., Alt, N., Somoza, V. and Lecerf, J. M., A diet based on high-heat-treated foods promotes risk factors for diabetes mellitus and cardiovascular diseases, Am J Clin Nutr, 91: 1220-1226.

4 Schalkwijk, C. G., Stehouwer, C. D. and van Hinsbergh, V. W., Fructose-mediated non-enzymatic glycation: sweet coupling or bad modification, Diabetes Metab Res Rev, 2004, 20: 369-382.

5 O'Brien, J. and Morrissey, P. A., Nutritional and toxicological aspects of the Maillard browning reaction in foods, Crit Rev Food Sci Nutr, 1989, 28: 211-248.

6 Sandu, O., Song, K., Cai, W., Zheng, F., Uribarri, J. and Vlassara, H., Insulin resistance and type 2 diabetes in high-fat-fed mice are linked to high glycotoxin intake, Diabetes, 2005, 54: 2314-2319.

6 Ding, J., Kritchevsky, S. B., Hsu, F. C., Harris, T. B., Burke, G. L., Detrano, R. C., Szklo, M., Criqui, M. H., Allison, M., Ouyang, P., Brown, E. R. and Carr, J. J., Association between non-subcutaneous adiposity and calcified coronary plaque: a substudy of the Multi-Ethnic Study of Atherosclerosis, Am J Clin Nutr, 2008, 88: 645-650.

7 Executive Summary of The Third Report of The National Cholesterol Education Program (NCEP) Expert Panel on Detection, Evaluation, And Treatment of High Blood Cholesterol In Adults (Adult Treatment Panel III), Jama, 2001, 285: 2486-2497.

8 Ford, E. S., Giles, W. H. and Dietz, W. H., Prevalence of the metabolic syndrome among US adults: findings from the third National Health and Nutrition Examination Survey, Jama, 2002, 287: 356-359.

9 Vlassara, H. and Striker, G., Glycotoxins in the diet promote diabetes and diabetic complications, Curr Diab Rep, 2007, 7: 235-241.

10 Hibbeln, J. R., Nieminen, L. R., Blasbalg, T. L., Riggs, J. A. and Lands, W. E., Healthy intakes of n-3 and n-6 fatty acids: estimations considering worldwide diversity, Am J Clin Nutr, 2006, 83: 1483S-1493S.

11 Kris-Etherton, P. M., Taylor, D. S., Yu-Poth, S., Huth, P., Moriarty, K., Fishell, V., Hargrove, R. L., Zhao, G. and Etherton, T. D., Polyunsaturated fatty acids in the food chain in the United States, Am J Clin Nutr, 2000, 71: 179S-188S.

12 Pischon, T., Hankinson, S. E., Hotamisligil, G. S., Rifai, N., Willett, W. C. and Rimm, E. B., Habitual dietary intake of n-3 and n-6 fatty acids in relation to inflammatory markers among US men and women, Circulation, 2003, 108: 155-160.

13 Willett, W. C., Diet and health: what should we eat?, Science, 1994, 264: 532-537

CHAPTER 4:

1   Dandona, P., Aljada, A., Chaudhuri, A., Mohanty, P. and Garg, R., Metabolic syndrome: a comprehensive perspective based on interactions between obesity, diabetes, and inflammation, Circulation, 2005, 111: 1448-1454.

2   Ford, E. S., Risks for all-cause mortality, cardiovascular disease, and diabetes associated with the metabolic syndrome: a summary of the evidence, Diabetes Care, 2005, 28: 1769-1778.

3   Knip, M., Veijola, R., Virtanen, S. M., Hyoty, H., Vaarala, O. and Akerblom, H. K., Environmental triggers and determinants of type 1 diabetes, Diabetes, 2005, 54 Suppl 2: S125-136.

4   Wentworth, J. M., Fourlanos, S. and Harrison, L. C., Reappraising the stereotypes of diabetes in the modern diabetogenic environment, Nat Rev Endocrinol, 2009, 5: 483-489.

5   Nathan, C., Epidemic inflammation: pondering obesity, Mol Med, 2008, 14: 485-492.

6   Riccardi, G., Giacco, R. and Rivellese, A. A., Dietary fat, insulin sensitivity and the metabolic syndrome, Clin Nutr, 2004, 23: 447-456.

7   Malik, V. S., Popkin, B. M., Bray, G. A., Despres, J. P. and Hu, F. B., Sugar-sweetened beverages, obesity, type 2 diabetes mellitus, and cardiovascular disease risk, Circulation, 2010, 121: 1356-1364.

9 Feuerer, M., Herrero, L., Cipolletta, D., Naaz, A., Wong, J., Nayer, A., Lee, J., Goldfine, A. B., Benoist, C., Shoelson, S. and Mathis, D., Lean, but not obese, fat is enriched for a unique population of regulatory T cells that affect metabolic parameters, Nat Med, 2009, 15: 930-939.

10 Shoelson, S. E., Lee, J. and Goldfine, A. B., Inflammation and insulin resistance, J Clin Invest, 2006, 116: 1793-1801.

11 Vlassara, H., Cai, W., Crandall, J., Goldberg, T., Oberstein, R., Dardaine, V., Peppa, M. and Rayfield, E. J., Inflammatory mediators are induced by dietary glycotoxins, a major risk factor for diabetic angiopathy, Proc Natl Acad Sci U S A, 2002, 99: 15596-15601.

12 Uribarri, J., Cai, Weijing, Ramdas, M, Goodman, S, Pyzik, R, Chen, L, Zu, L, Striker, G, Vlassara, H, Improved insulin resistance in human type 2 diabetes by advanced glycosylation end product restriction, Diabetes Care, 2011, 34: 1-7.

13 Fraley, A. E., Schwartz, G. G., Olsson, A. G., Kinlay, S., Szarek, M., Rifai, N., Libby, P., Ganz, P., Witztum, J. L. and Tsimikas, S., Relationship of oxidized phospholipids and biomarkers of oxidized low-density lipoprotein with cardiovascular risk factors, inflammatory biomarkers, and effect of statin therapy in patients with acute coronary syndromes: Results from the MIRACL (Myocardial Ischemia Reduction With Aggressive Cholesterol Lowering) trial, J Am Coll Cardiol, 2009, 53: 2186-2196.

14 Camhi, S. M., Understanding potential mechanisms linking low-fat diet to inflammation and metabolic syndrome, Metabolism, 2010, 59: 455-456.

15 Camhi, S. M., Stefanick, M. L., Ridker, P. M. and Young, D. R., Changes in C-reactive protein from low-fat diet and/or physical activity in men and women with and without metabolic syndrome, Metabolism, 2010, 59: 54-61.

16 Lin, R. Y., Choudhury, R. P., Cai, W., Lu, M., Fallon, J. T., Fisher, E. A. and Vlassara, H., Dietary glycotoxins promote diabetic atherosclerosis in apolipoprotein E-deficient mice, Atherosclerosis, 2003, 168: 213-220.

17 Stirban, A., Negrean, M., Stratmann, B., Gawlowski, T., Horstmann, T., Gotting, C., Kleesiek, K., Mueller-Roesel, M., Koschinsky, T., Uribarri, J., Vlassara, H. and Tschoepe, D., Benfotiamine prevents macro- and microvascular endothelial dysfunction and oxidative stress following a meal rich in advanced glycation end products in individuals with type 2 diabetes, Diabetes Care, 2006, 29: 2064-2071.

18 Uribarri, J., Stirban, A., Sander, D., Cai, W., Negrean, M., Buenting, C. E., Koschinsky, T. and Vlassara, H., Single oral challenge by advanced glycation end products acutely impairs endothelial function in diabetic and nondiabetic subjects, Diabetes Care, 2007, 30: 2579-2582.

20 Makita, Z., Radoff, S., Rayfield, E. J., Yang, Z., Skolnik, E., Delaney, V., Friedman, E. A., Cerami, A. and Vlassara, H., Advanced glycosylation end products in patients with diabetic nephropathy, N Engl J Med, 1991, 325: 836-842.

24 Vlassara, H., Striker, L. J., Teichberg, S., Fuh, H., Li, Y. M. and Steffes, M., Advanced glycation end products induce glomerular sclerosis and albuminuria in normal rats, Proc Natl Acad Sci U S A, 1994, 91: 11704-11708.

25 Vlassara, H., Torreggiani, M., Post, J. B., Zheng, F., Uribarri, J. and Striker, G. E., Role of oxidants/inflammation in declining renal function in chronic kidney disease and normal aging, Kidney Int Suppl, 2009: S3-11.

26 Vlassara, H., Striker, GE,, Diabetes and AGEs, A New Paradigm and Indications, Nature Endocrinology, 2011, in press.

27 Despres, J. P. and Lemieux, I., Abdominal obesity and metabolic syndrome, Nature, 2006, 444: 881-887.

28 Despres, J. P. and Lemieux, I., Abdominal obesity and metabolic syndrome, Nature, 2006, 444: 881-887.

29 Delahanty, L. M., Nathan, D. M., Lachin, J. M., Hu, F. B., Cleary, P. A., Ziegler, G. K., Wylie-Rosett, J. and Wexler, D. J., Association of diet with glycated hemoglobin during intensive treatment of type 1 diabetes in the Diabetes Control and Complications Trial, Am J Clin Nutr, 2009, 89: 518-524.

30 Schwartz, A. V., Vittinghoff, E., Sellmeyer, D. E., Feingold, K. R., de Rekeneire, N., Strotmeyer, E. S., Shorr, R. I., Vinik, A. I., Odden, M. C., Park, S. W., Faulkner, K. A. and Harris, T. B., Diabetes-related complications, glycemic control, and falls in older adults, Diabetes Care, 2008, 31: 391-396.

31 Young, B. A., Lin, E., Von Korff, M., Simon, G., Ciechanowski, P., Ludman, E. J., Everson-Stewart, S., Kinder, L., Oliver, M., Boyko, E. J. and Katon, W. J., Diabetes complications severity index and risk of mortality, hospitalization, and healthcare utilization, Am J Manag Care, 2008, 14: 15-23.

32 Staessen, J. A., Can lowering blood pressure prevent vascular complications in patients with type 2 diabetes?, Nat Clin Pract Cardiovasc Med, 2008, 5: 194-195.

33 Tomlin, A. M., Dovey, S. M. and Tilyard, M. W., Risk factors for hospitalization due to diabetes complications, Diabetes Res Clin Pract, 2008, 80: 244-252.

34 Peppa, M., He, C., Hattori, M., McEvoy, R., Zheng, F. and Vlassara, H., Fetal or neonatal low-glycotoxin environment prevents autoimmune diabetes in NOD mice, Diabetes, 2003, 52: 1441-1448.

35 Coresh, J., Byrd-Holt, D., Astor, B. C., Briggs, J. P., Eggers, P. W., Lacher, D. A. and Hostetter, T. H., Chronic kidney disease awareness, prevalence, and trends among U.S. adults, 1999 to 2000, J Am Soc Nephrol, 2005, 16: 180-188.

36 Perkovic, V., Verdon, C., Ninomiya, T., Barzi, F., Cass, A., Patel, A., Jardine, M., Gallagher, M., Turnbull, F., Chalmers, J., Craig, J. and Huxley, R., The relationship between proteinuria and coronary risk: a systematic review and meta-analysis, PLoS Med, 2008, 5: e207.

39 Erten-Lyons, D., Woltjer, R. L., Dodge, H., Nixon, R., Vorobik, R., Calvert, J. F., Leahy, M., Montine, T. and Kaye, J., Factors associated with resistance to dementia despite high Alzheimer disease pathology, Neurology, 2009, 72: 354-360.

40 Sato, T., Shimogaito, N., Wu, X., Kikuchi, S., Yamagishi, S. and Takeuchi, M., Toxic advanced glycation end products (TAGE)

theory in Alzheimer's disease, Am J Alzheimers Dis Other Demen, 2006, 21: 197-208.

41 Takeuchi, M. and Yamagishi, S., Possible involvement of advanced glycation end-products (AGEs) in the pathogenesis of Alzheimer's disease, Curr Pharm Des, 2008, 14: 973-978.

42 Zheng, F., He, C., Cai, W., Hattori, M., Steffes, M. and Vlassara, H., Prevention of diabetic nephropathy in mice by a diet low in glycoxidation products, Diabetes Metab Res Rev, 2002, 18: 224-237.

43 Holvoet, P., Mertens, A., Verhamme, P., Bogaerts, K., Beyens, G., Verhaeghe, R., Collen, D., Muls, E. and Van de Werf, F., Circulating oxidized LDL is a useful marker for identifying patients with coronary artery disease, Arterioscler Thromb Vasc Biol, 2001, 21: 844-848.

CHAPTER 5:

1. Caleb E. Finch, The Biology of Human longevity, Academic Press, 2007

2. Longo, V. D. and Finch, C. E., Evolutionary medicine: from dwarf model systems to healthy centenarians?, Science, 2003, 299: 1342-1346.

3. Lapointe, J. and Hekimi, S., When a theory of aging ages badly, Cell Mol Life Sci, 2010, 67: 1-8.

4. Vlassara, H., Fuh, H., Makita, Z., Krungkrai, S., Cerami, A. and Bucala, R., Exogenous advanced glycosylation end products induce complex vascular dysfunction in normal animals: a model for diabetic and aging complications, Proc Natl Acad Sci U S A, 1992, 89: 12043-12047.

5. Semba, R. D., Bandinelli, S., Sun, K., Guralnik, J. M. and Ferrucci, L., Plasma carboxymethyl-lysine, an advanced glycation end product, and all-cause and cardiovascular disease mortality in older community-dwelling adults, J Am Geriatr Soc, 2009, 57: 1874-1880.

6. Fontana, L. and Klein, S., Aging, adiposity, and calorie restriction, Jama, 2007, 297: 986-994.

7. Fontana, L., Klein, S. and Holloszy, J. O., Long-term low-protein, low-calorie diet and endurance exercise modulate metabolic factors associated with cancer risk, Am J Clin Nutr, 2006, 84: 1456-1462.

8. Cai, W., He, J. C., Zhu, L., Chen, X., Zheng, F., Striker, G. E. and Vlassara, H., Oral glycotoxins determine the effects of calorie restriction on oxidant stress, age-related diseases, and lifespan, Am J Pathol, 2008, 173: 327-336.

9. Weil, A., Healthy Aging, New York, 2007.

10. Uribarri, J., Cai, W., Peppa, M., Goodman, S., Ferrucci, L., Striker, G. and Vlassara, H., Circulating glycotoxins and dietary advanced glycation endproducts: two links to inflammatory response, oxidative stress, and aging, J Gerontol A Biol Sci Med Sci, 2007, 62: 427-433.

11. Krishnan, S. T., Quattrini, C., Jeziorska, M., Malik, R. A. and Rayman, G., Neurovascular factors in wound healing in the foot skin of type 2 diabetic subjects, Diabetes Care, 2007, 30: 3058-3062.

12. Welsh-Bohmer, K. A. and White, C. L., 3rd, Alzheimer disease: what changes in the brain cause dementia?, Neurology, 2009, 72: e21.

13. Vitek, M. P., Bhattacharya, K., Glendening, J. M., Stopa, E., Vlassara, H., Bucala, R., Manogue, K. and Cerami, A., Advanced glycation end products contribute to amyloidosis in Alzheimer disease, Proc Natl Acad Sci U S A, 1994, 91: 4766-4770.

14. Munch, G., Schinzel, R., Loske, C., Wong, A., Durany, N., Li, J. J., Vlassara, H., Smith, M. A., Perry, G. and Riederer, P., Alzheimer's disease–synergistic effects of glucose deficit, oxidative stress and advanced glycation endproducts, J Neural Transm, 1998, 105: 439-461

15. Bar, K. J., Franke, S., Wenda, B., Muller, S., Kientsch-Engel, R., Stein, G. and Sauer, H., Pentosidine and

N(epsilon)-(carboxymethyl)-lysine in Alzheimer's disease and vascular dementia, Neurobiol Aging, 2003, 24: 333-338.

16 Luchsinger, J. A., Tang, M. X., Shea, S. and Mayeux, R., Hyperinsulinemia and risk of Alzheimer disease, Neurology, 2004, 63: 1187-1192.

17 Luchsinger, J. A. and Mayeux, R., Dietary factors and Alzheimer's disease, Lancet Neurol, 2004, 3: 579-587.

18 Luchsinger, J. A. and Mayeux, R., Cardiovascular risk factors and Alzheimer's disease, Curr Atheroscler Rep, 2004, 6: 261-266.

19 Zimmerman, G. A., Meistrell, M., 3rd, Bloom, O., Cockroft, K. M., Bianchi, M., Risucci, D., Broome, J., Farmer, P., Cerami, A., Vlassara, H. and et al., Neurotoxicity of advanced glycation endproducts during focal stroke and neuroprotective effects of aminoguanidine, Proc Natl Acad Sci U S A, 1995, 92: 3744-3748.

20 Fan, X., Zhang, J., Theves, M., Strauch, C., Nemet, I., Liu, X., Qian, J., Giblin, F. J. and Monnier, V. M., Mechanism of lysine oxidation in human lens crystallins during aging and in diabetes, J Biol Chem, 2009, 284: 34618-34627.

21 Monnier, V. M., Bautista, O., Kenny, D., Sell, D. R., Fogarty, J., Dahms, W., Cleary, P. A., Lachin, J. and Genuth, S., Skin collagen glycation, glycoxidation, and crosslinking are lower in subjects with long-term intensive versus conventional therapy of type 1 diabetes: relevance of glycated collagen products versus HbA1c as markers of diabetic complications. DCCT Skin Collagen Ancillary Study Group. Diabetes Control and Complications Trial, Diabetes, 1999, 48: 870-880.

22 Peppa, M., Brem, H., Ehrlich, P., Zhang, J. G., Cai, W., Li, Z., Croitoru, A., Thung, S. and Vlassara, H., Adverse effects of dietary glycotoxins on wound healing in genetically diabetic mice, Diabetes, 2003, 52: 2805-2813.

23 Sell, D. R., Lapolla, A., Odetti, P., Fogarty, J. and Monnier, V. M., Pentosidine formation in skin correlates with severity of complications in individuals with long-standing IDDM, Diabetes, 1992, 41: 1286-1292.

24 Genuth, S., Sun, W., Cleary, P., Sell, D. R., Dahms, W., Malone, J., Sivitz, W. and Monnier, V. M., Glycation and carboxymethyl-lysine levels in skin collagen predict the risk of future 10-year progression of diabetic retinopathy and nephropathy in the diabetes control and complications trial and epidemiology of diabetes interventions and complications participants with type 1 diabetes, Diabetes, 2005, 54: 3103-3111.

25 Cerami, C., Founds, H., Nicholl, I., Mitsuhashi, T., Giordano, D., Vanpatten, S., Lee, A., Al-Abed, Y., Vlassara, H., Bucala, R. and Cerami, A., Tobacco smoke is a source of toxic reactive glycation products, Proc Natl Acad Sci U S A, 1997, 94: 13915-13920.

26 Shahinfar, S., Dickson, T. Z., Ahmed, T., Zhang, Z., Ramjit, D., Smith, R. D. and Brenner, B. M., Losartan in patients with type 2 diabetes and proteinuria: observations from the RENAAL Study, Kidney Int Suppl, 2002: S64-67.

12 Olshansky, S. J., Passaro, D. J., Hershow, R. C., Layden, J., Carnes, B. A., Brody, J., Hayflick, L., Butler, R. N., Allison, D. B. and Ludwig, D. S., A potential decline in life expectancy in the United States in the 21st century, N Engl J Med, 2005, 352: 1138-1145.

16 Trichopoulou, A. and Vasilopoulou, E., Mediterranean diet and longevity, Br J Nutr, 2000, 84 Suppl 2: S205-209.

CHAPTER 6:

1 Clerisme-Beaty, E. and Rand, C. S., The effect of obesity on asthma incidence: moving past the epidemiologic evidence, J Allergy Clin Immunol, 2009, 123: 96-97.

2 Fourlanos, S., Harrison, L. C. and Colman, P. G., The accelerator hypothesis and increasing incidence of type 1 diabetes, Curr Opin Endocrinol Diabetes Obes, 2008, 15: 321-325.

3 Birlouez-Aragon, I., Pischetsrieder, M., Leclere, J., Morales, F.J., Hasenkopf, K., Kientsch-Engel, R., Ducauze, C.J., Rutledge, D., Assessment of protein glycation markers in infant formulas, Food Chemistry, 2004, 87: 253-259.

4   Zutavern, A., Brockow, I., Schaaf, B., von Berg, A., Diez, U., Borte, M., Kraemer, U., Herbarth, O., Behrendt, H., Wichmann, H. E. and Heinrich, J., Timing of solid food introduction in relation to eczema, asthma, allergic rhinitis, and food and inhalant sensitization at the age of 6 years: results from the prospective birth cohort study LISA, Pediatrics, 2008, 121: e44-52.
5   Mericq, V., Piccardo, C., Cai, W., Chen, X., Zhu, L., Striker, G. E., Vlassara, H. and Uribarri, J., Maternally transmitted and food-derived glycotoxins: a factor preconditioning the young to diabetes?, Diabetes Care, 2010, 33: 2232-2237.
6   Schmid, R., The Untold Story of Milk, Washington, D.C., New Trends Publishing, Inc., 2007.

CHAPTER 7:

1   Makita, Z., Vlassara, H., Cerami, A. and Bucala, R., Immunochemical detection of advanced glycosylation end products in vivo, J Biol Chem, 1992, 267: 5133-5138.
2   Makita, Z., Vlassara, H., Rayfield, E., Cartwright, K., Friedman, E., Rodby, R., Cerami, A. and Bucala, R., Hemoglobin-AGE: a circulating marker of advanced glycosylation, Science, 1992, 258: 651-653.
3   Semba, R. D., Bandinelli, S., Sun, K., Guralnik, J. M. and Ferrucci, L., Plasma carboxymethyl-lysine, an advanced glycation end product, and all-cause and cardiovascular disease mortality in older community-dwelling adults, J Am Geriatr Soc, 2009, 57: 1874-1880.
4   Onorato, J. M., Jenkins, A. J., Thorpe, S. R. and Baynes, J. W., Pyridoxamine, an inhibitor of advanced glycation reactions, also inhibits advanced lipoxidation reactions. Mechanism of action of pyridoxamine, J Biol Chem, 2000, 275: 21177-21184.
5   Du, X., Edelstein, D. and Brownlee, M., Oral benfotiamine plus alpha-lipoic acid normalises complication-causing pathways in type 1 diabetes, Diabetologia, 2008, 51: 1930-1932.

6   Mitsuhashi, T., Vlassara, H., Founds, H. W. and Li, Y. M., Standardizing the immunological measurement of advanced glycation endproducts using normal human serum, J Immunol Methods, 1997, 207: 79-88.

7   Radoff, S., Makita, Z. and Vlassara, H., Radioreceptor assay for advanced glycosylation end products, Diabetes, 1991, 40: 1731-1738.

8   Makita, Z., Vlassara, H., Rayfield, E., Cartwright, K., Friedman, E., Rodby, R., Cerami, A. and Bucala, R., Hemoglobin-AGE: a circulating marker of advanced glycosylation, Science, 1992, 258: 651-653.

9   Li, Y. M., Steffes, M., Donnelly, T., Liu, C., Fuh, H., Basgen, J., Bucala, R. and Vlassara, H., Prevention of cardiovascular and renal pathology of aging by the advanced glycation inhibitor aminoguanidine, Proc Natl Acad Sci U S A, 1996, 93: 3902-3907.

10 USDA, Food Supply Trends: More Calories, Refined Carbohydrates and Calories, Food Review, 1999, 22.3.

CHAPTER 8:

1   Floyd, C. H., the Gene Smart Diet, Rodale, 2009

2   Schmid, R., The Untold Story of Milk, Washington, D.C., New Trends Publishing, Inc., 2007.

3   Perren, R., Structural Change and Market Growth in the Food Industry: Flour Milling in Britain, Europe, and America, 1850-1914., 1990.

4   Trichopoulou, A. and Vasilopoulou, E., Mediterranean diet and longevity, Br J Nutr, 2000, 84 Suppl 2: S205-209.

5   Nestle, M., Real Food: What to Eat New York, North Point Press, 2006.

6   Simopoulos, A., The Mediterranean Diets: What is so Special About the Diet of Greece? The Scientific Evidence, In, American Institute for Cancer Research 11th Annual Research Conference on Diet, Nutrition and Cancer, Washington, DC, Journal of Nutrition, 2001.

Made in the USA
Charleston, SC
25 September 2013